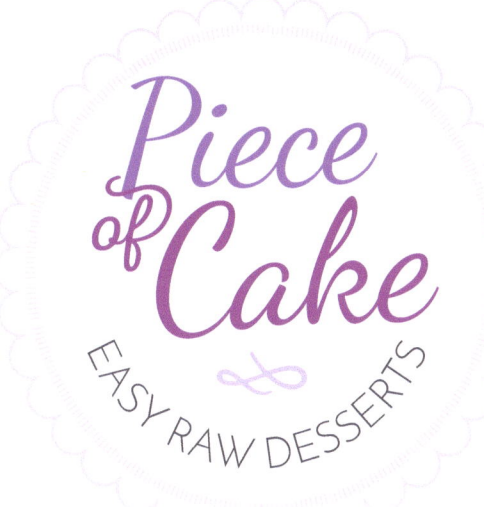

Natalie Prigoone

Copyright © 2016 by Natalie Prigoone

All rights reserved. This book or any portion thereof may not be reproduced or used in any manner whatsoever without the express written permission of the publisher except for the use of brief quotations in a book review.

For permission requests, write to the publisher, addressed "Attention: Permissions Coordinator," at natalieprigoone@gmail.com

Thirsty Knowledge Publishing

www.thegreatuncooking.com

First Published, 2016

Author: Prigoone, Natalie.

Title: Piece of Cake: Easy Raw Desserts

ISBN: 978-0-9945955-0-8

Subjects: Cooking (Natural foods), Desserts, Raw food diet, Health.

Book Designed by: Lisa Valuyskaya www.ideastylist.com

Food photographed and styled by: Natalie Prigoone. www.rawfoodrecipes.co

Author photo by: Jesse Smith www.jessesmith.com.au

This book is not intended as a substitute for the medical advice of physicians. The reader should regularly consult a physician in matters relating to his/ her health and particularly with respect to any symptoms that may require diagnosis, medical attention or a special diet.

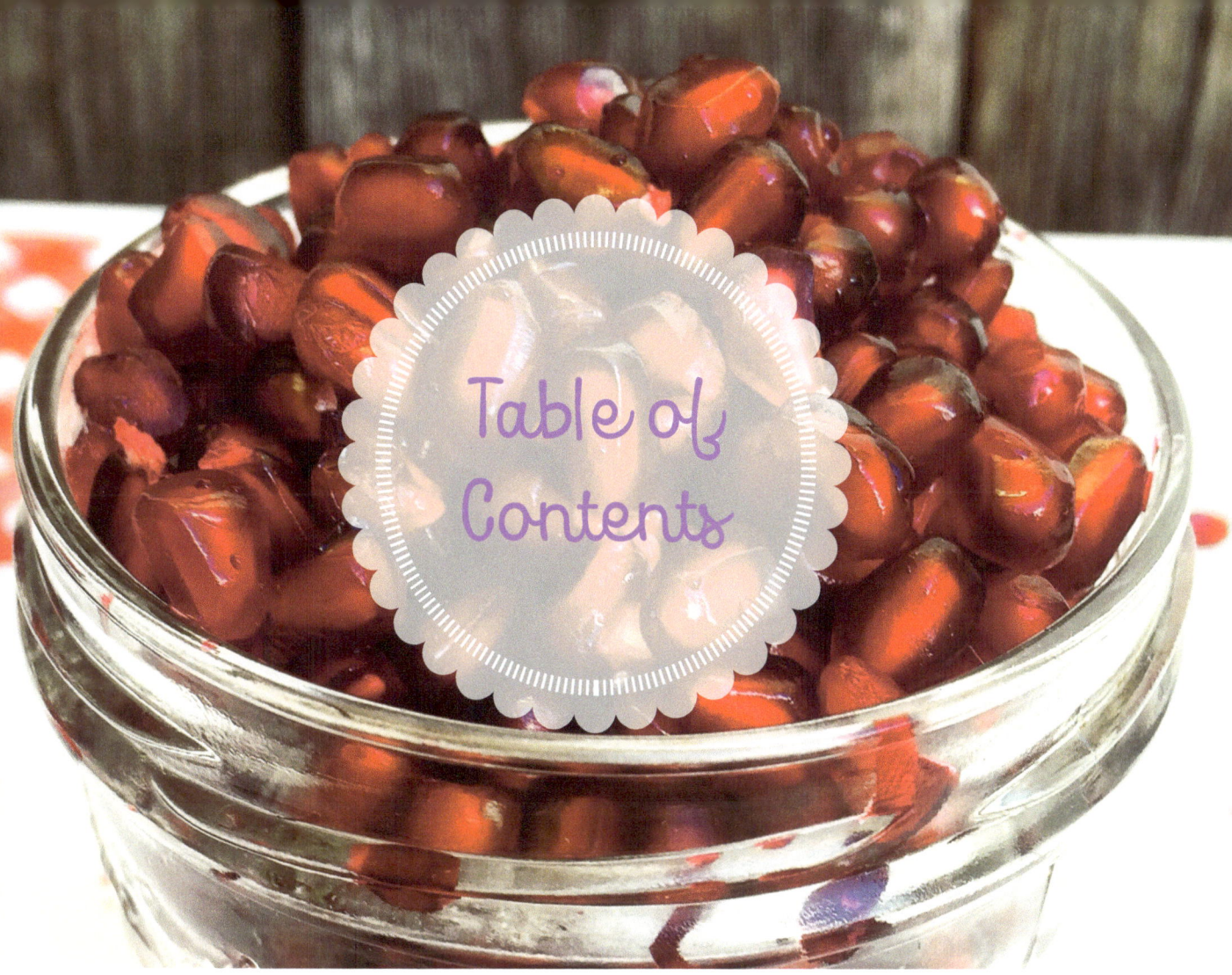

Table of Contents

Introduction 4
Tools of the Trade 8
The Basics: Life Without Sugar, Dairy or Wheat Flour 10
Recipes 16
Ice-creams 18
Cheesecakes 42
Chocolates and Fudge 72
Breakfast Desserts 90
Cookies, Slices and Energy Balls 102
Thank you 126

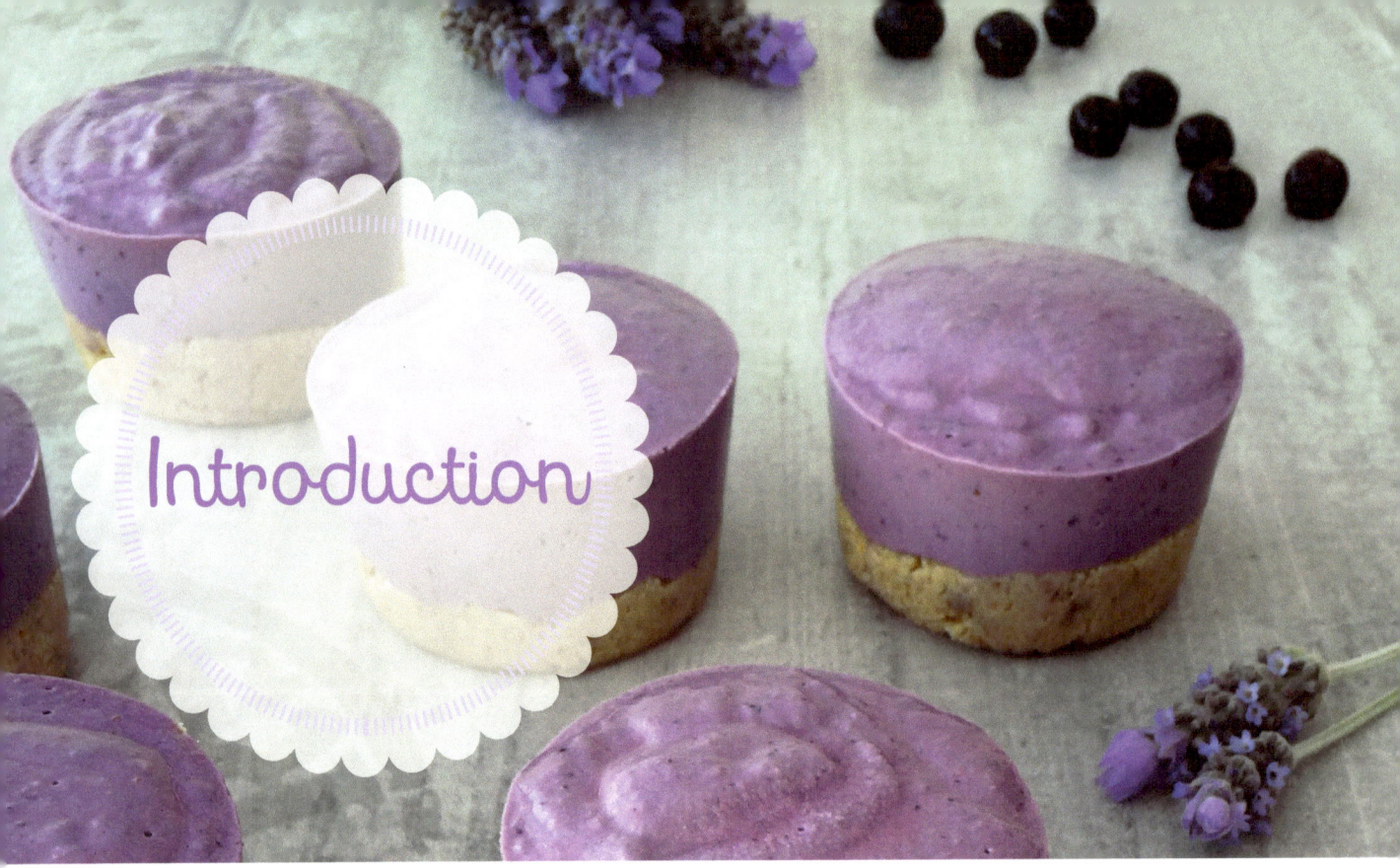

Introduction

DESSERTS AND WOMEN GO TOGETHER...

Yet go to a restaurant and you may hear a man complain that his female companion wants to share his dessert, even though she declined ordering her own. Heaven forbid! Why is this? Why, when women so obviously love desserts, do they forgo them when presented with an opportunity to have their own at the conclusion of a meal? Guilt may be one answer, wanting to watch their figure may be another closely linked, and now we have the scientific community warning us of the perils of sugar and the links to cancer. It is with these things in mind that I have created nourishing dessert recipes that are free from refined addiction-forming sugar, wheat and dairy, and free from guilt.

GUILT FREE DESSERTS?

Yes, all these recipes can be enjoyed without guilt because you won't be doing something bad to your body. They are, however, still treats. *Vegetables* should form the main part of our diet, and *these recipes are not vegetables.* They are however, plant-based. Because these desserts are nutrient dense, a little goes a long way. They are rich, delicious and satiating. This means you won't feel compelled to eat a whole cake in one sitting.

You can quite easily store these desserts in the freezer and pull them out when the sweet cravings hit. In fact, part of embracing a healthy life involves being prepared with healthy alternatives for when our resolve is low and our cravings high. Have a stash of peanut protein balls on hand in the fridge or freezer, or perhaps some peppermint super-food chocolates. That way when you are reaching for a treat it will be one that is both nourishing and satisfying.

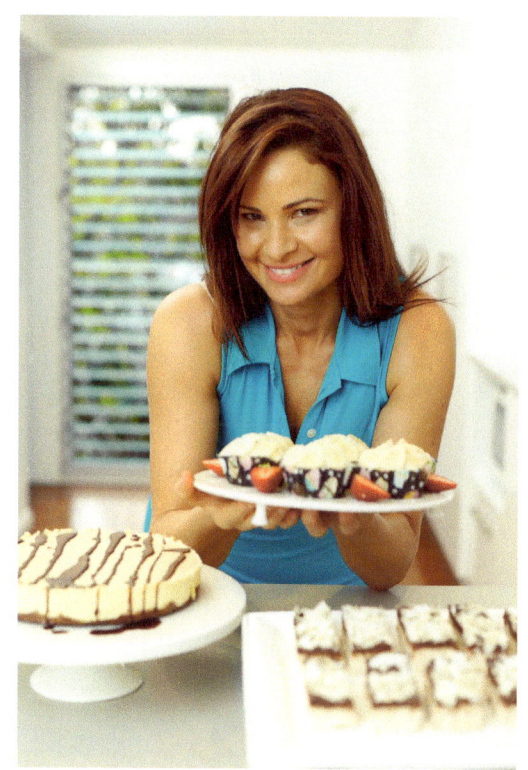

Why Raw Vegan Desserts?

Raw desserts are suitable for anyone who is following a vegetarian, vegan, paleo, or raw food diet. It's awesome for anyone who can't have dairy or grains and it's especially great if you are trying to cut out processed sugars. Basically, they are great for anyone.

NO BAKE

Raw means not cooked. All the nuts used in these recipes are raw – not roasted. Check the labels before you purchase your nuts. Raw cacao powder is used instead of roasted cocoa powder. From time to time an oven or dehydrator may be used on a low temperature to dry out some foods. There is no baking. Most things require a good blender or food processor. It's pretty hard to make a mistake. Unlike traditional baking which can fail you if you are not exact, raw food preparation is forgiving.

Tips

There are a few tricks I use that make my recipes taste awesome. Firstly, I boost the sweetness with stevia. This doesn't add any further calories. I don't use this sweetener exclusively because it doesn't taste pleasant in large quantities and it doesn't provide volume or the viscous properties that syrups such as rice malt or maple syrup have.

Secondly, I like to boost flavor with culinary essential oils. Think of these oils as the filter that boosts color on your Instagram photos. While they aren't essential, they 'value add' to flavour. You can always just add more lime and more rice malt syrup, (or whatever the recipe calls for), tasting as you go; adjusting the sweetness and flavor to your liking. If it's been some time since you've had sugary foods, then your palate will be more sensitive to the sweetness and will require less sweetener.

Know the difference between coconut paste and coconut oil. Coconut paste is the ground down mature coconut flesh. I use both in these recipes for different effects. Sometimes you can replace the coconut paste with coconut oil but not in the fudge or bounty bar recipes. In those recipes, the coconut paste is a key ingredient.

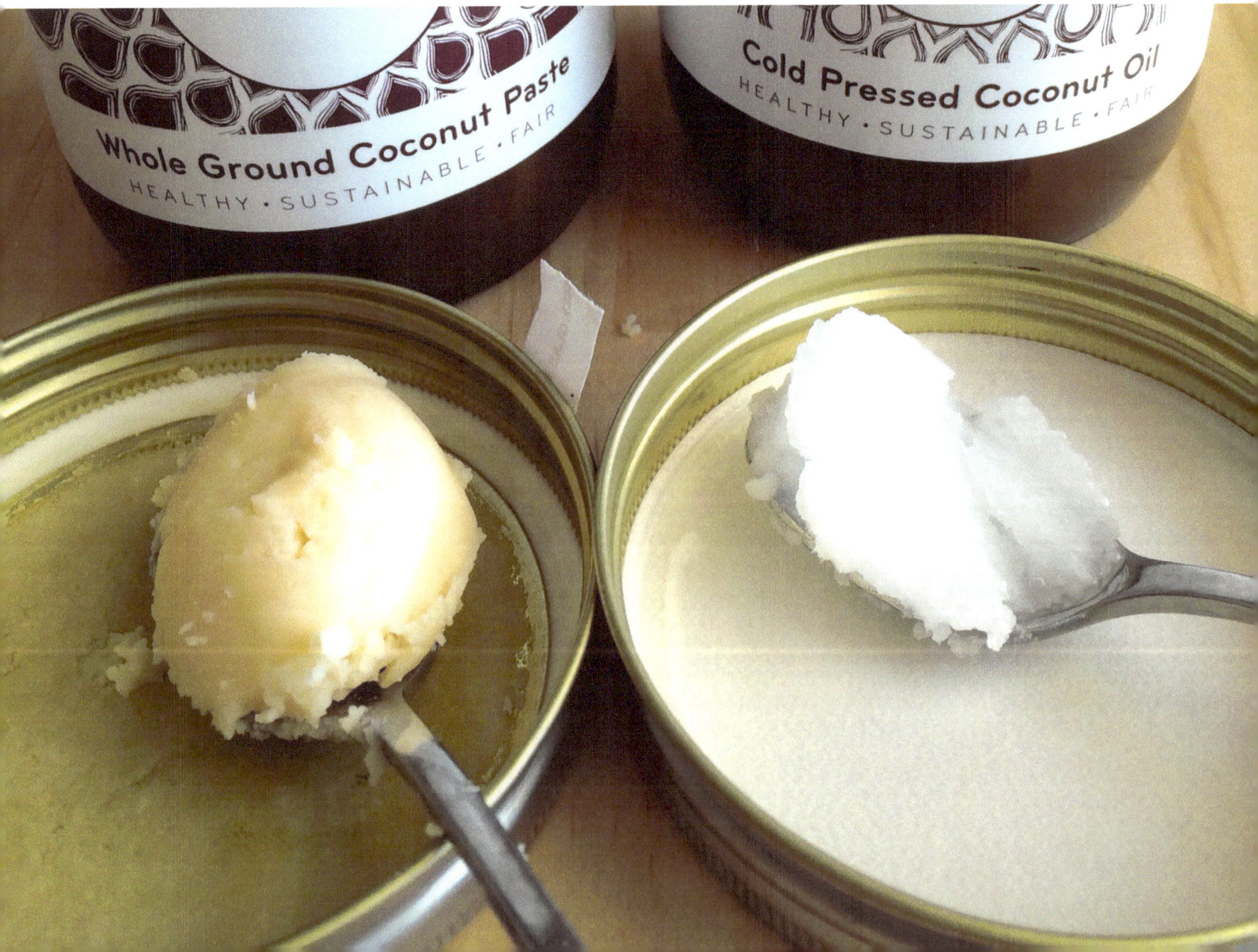

A NOTE ABOUT MELTING:

Use a bowl of hot water then place your cacao butter or coconut paste/oil in a dish or glass jar resting in the bowl of hot water. Make sure you don't use a microwave or it will make your expensive raw ingredients not raw and lose their healing magic.

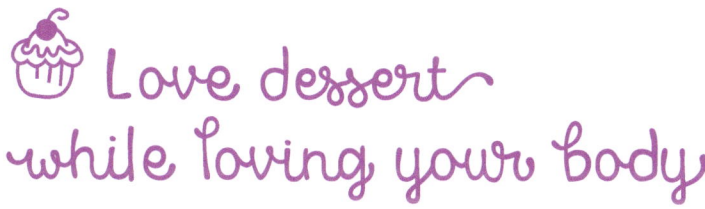

Love dessert while loving your body

It's important psychologically and socially to indulge in a little celebratory dessert now and then. I would argue that it's even a must for staying on the healthy eating path. So I bring to you a collection of some of my desserts for you to make or be inspired by to reinvent your own favorites. These treats are still full of calories because they are nutrient dense. They will feed your cells, heal your body and allow for that amorous feeling we all get when we consume chocolate or creamy decadent treats.

However, these desserts are filling, satisfying and won't leave you feeling out of control. Listen to your body. Eat intuitively with the intention of nourishing your cells and you won't go wrong.

Above all, enjoy what you eat.

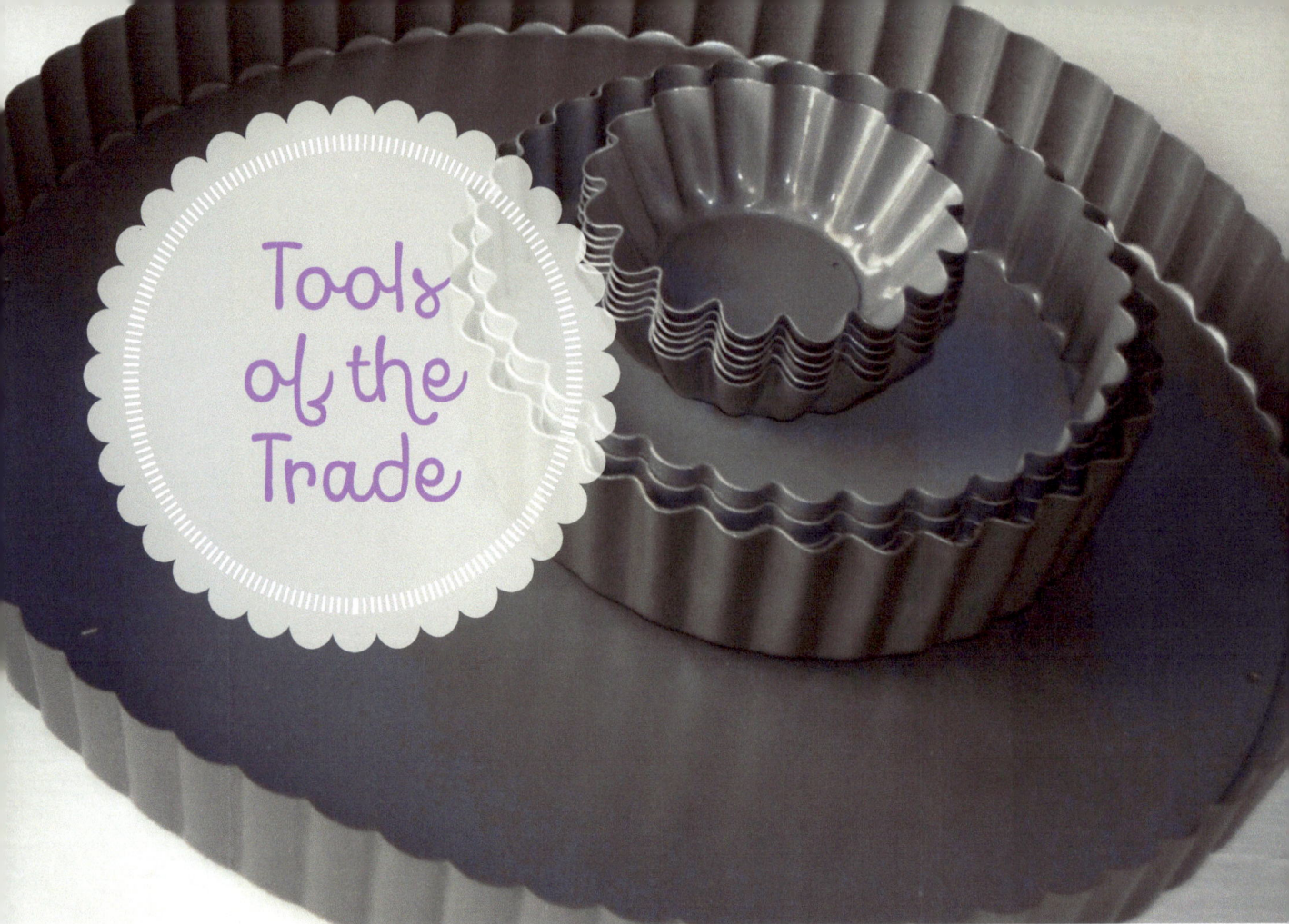

Tools of the Trade

The raw food cook needs a powerful blender and a food processor. Without these two tools you will find it difficult to make these recipes. You don't have to have a Thermomix or Vitamix (although they would be ideal), but another equally powerful processing machine would make life easier. There are many on the market. Choose one that has a warranty on the motor for 10 or 20 years. Then you know it's going to stand up to heavy-duty wear and tear.

The good news is that that's about all you need. Grab a handful of your favorite baking tins and cake pans and you are ready to go. I also find that a good supply of baking paper saves a lot of hassles.

Food processor with large bowl

Blender

Don't feel compelled to buy all these tins. Use what you have. Raw desserts are forgiving. It's not like baking, where depth of tin affects cooking time.

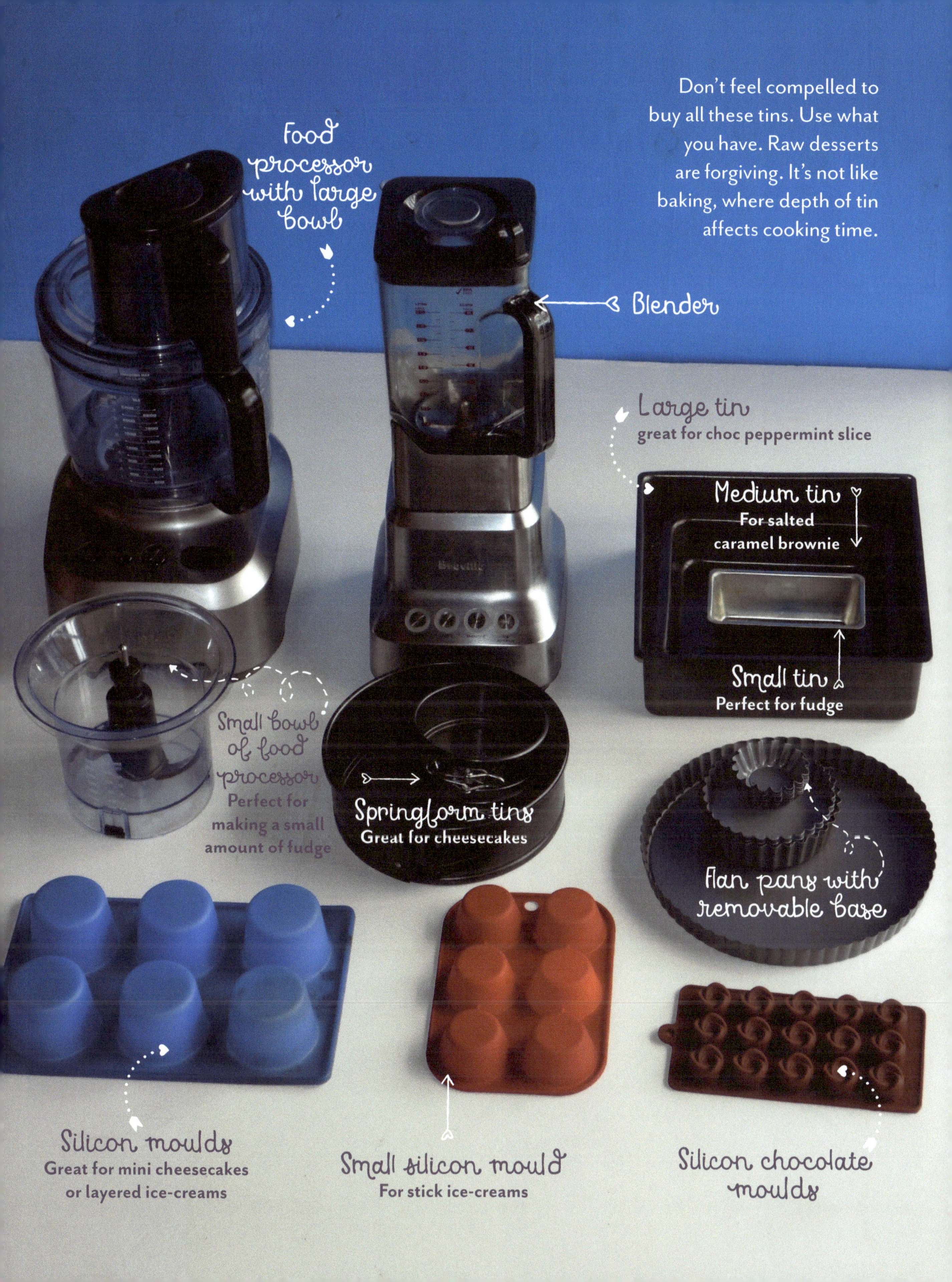

Large tin
great for choc peppermint slice

Medium tin
For salted caramel brownie

Small tin
Perfect for fudge

Small bowl of food processor
Perfect for making a small amount of fudge

Springform tins
Great for cheesecakes

Flan pans with removable base

Silicon moulds
Great for mini cheesecakes or layered ice-creams

Small silicon mould
For stick ice-creams

Silicon chocolate moulds

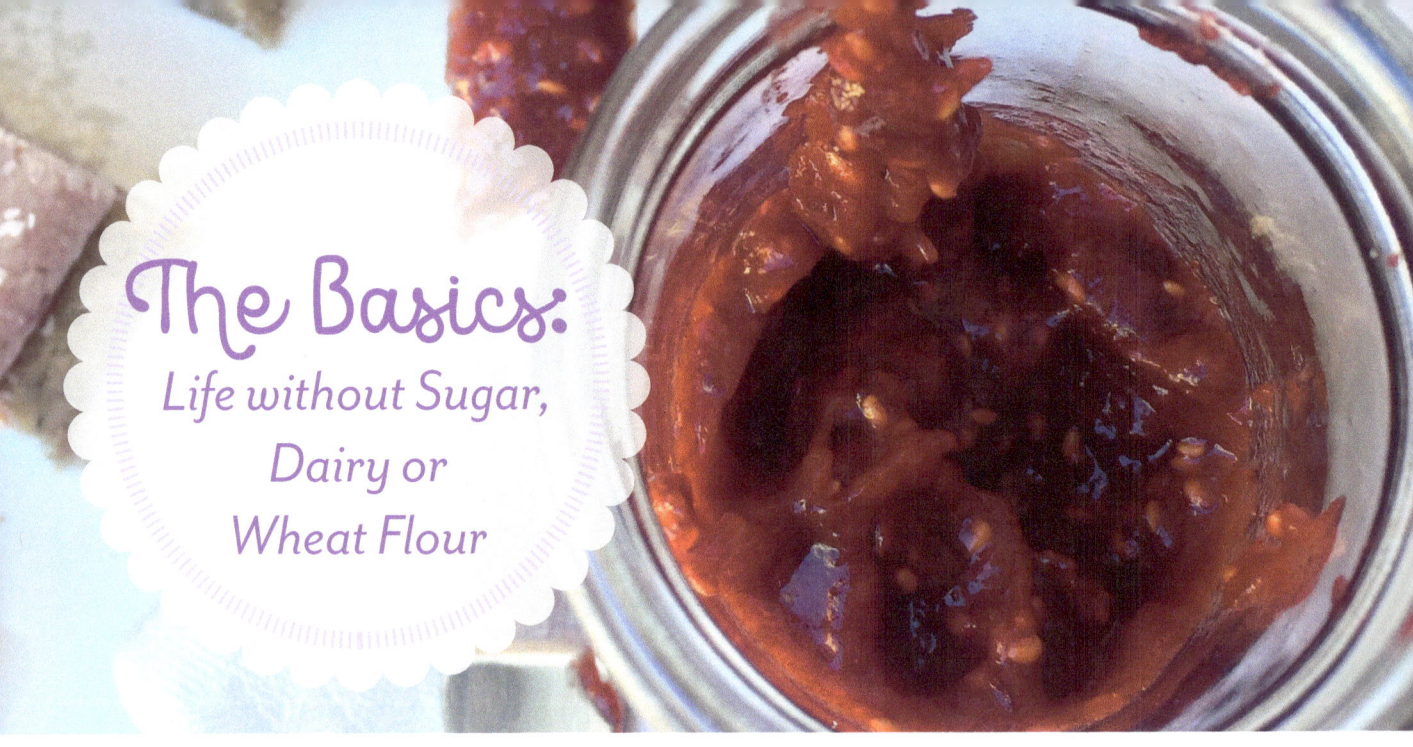

The Basics:
Life without Sugar, Dairy or Wheat Flour

I LOVE DESSERT.

You do too? Well, we are both in the right place. If you have a love of health, then you may have encountered some of the problems that I have met. Dessert and health are usually in opposition; or they were until now. Now there is a movement away from things that make us ill (sugar, wheat, dairy) and a reinvention of classic desserts and sweet treats into food that is nourishing. **Nourishing and delicious.**

I discovered that it is impossible for me to give up sweets. I've tried, but they make me happy. They make the people I share them with happy, and they really do release endorphins, the body's natural opiates. Desserts also look pretty and as the poem goes, "…little girls are made of sugar and spice and all things nice."

Most desserts are made of a combination of wheat, dairy, sugar and eggs. The challenge for a raw vegan chef is to create equally delicious desserts without using these ingredients. For a deeper explanation of why a raw foodist would omit these foods, see my first book "The Great Uncooking". Even though I revere the humble egg, for the purpose of delivering a book that is suitable for all I'm sticking to raw vegan principles.

Substitutions

SUGAR-FREE

This term implies that the food is free from added table sugar. But since a dessert that doesn't taste sweet is not really a dessert, we are going to have to use more healthful alternatives. We are trying to minimize the fructose sugars. If it's in a whole fruit, it's fine. The included fiber, minerals and vitamins make it completely healthful. These desserts will rely on some low or fructose free natural sweeteners.

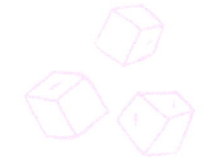

Stevia

Stevia is a great natural sweetener that has virtually no calories and no effect on the pancreas or blood glucose levels. However, because of its properties i.e., a distinctive aftertaste, low volume and low viscosity, it is not ideal as a simple replacement for syrups or sugar. As a rule, I try to use as little sweetener as possible, such as rice malt syrup and coconut flower syrup, and then boost with stevia. This way I can achieve the texture and volume that I need without altering the flavor of the dish I am creating.

Another thing to note about stevia is that it comes in a variety of concentrations and, because of this, it can be difficult to say exactly how much you should add. Read the label that should indicate how sweet it is compared to an equivalent tsp of sugar. I use vanilla stevia drops in smoothies and ice-creams when I just need to tweak the sweetness. I use both green and white powdered stevia. The green is less refined and more true to its origins as a green plant, but it does have a distinct flavor so it's best used in small amounts.

Maple Syrup

Maple syrup is a low fructose natural syrup that has a beautiful flavor. Its high liquid content makes it perfect for helping mixtures like chocolate to seize (set). Make sure you only buy 100% pure maple syrup and not the imitation variety that says 'maple flavored syrup".

Rice Malt Syrup

Rice malt syrup has a great neutral flavor. It adds sweetness without any real flavor. Its high viscosity and reluctance to freeze solid makes it the perfect choice when I want things to be soft and creamy, such as in ice-cream.

Coconut Flower Syrup

This is also known as coconut flower nectar. It has a lovely unique flavor and is nutritious. However, it is high in fructose. It can replace both rice malt and maple syrup in recipes, but use with caution.

Xylitol

Xylitol has a sugar-like texture that is granular or crystalline, making it difficult to dissolve at low temps. I use xylitol when I want sweetness with a course grainy dry texture, or a bit of a crunch. It's great for slices and cheesecake bases.

I don't use Agave. It has been used widely in many raw food recipes as a healthy alternative but it is very high in fructose (60 -65%, which makes it higher than high fructose corn syrup). Don't even go there! You'd be better off with honey which, Although high in fructose, is at least antiviral, antibacterial, antifungal and tasty.

GRAIN-FREE

Wheat flour is replaced with nut flours and nut blends. Gluten free flours made without wheat are also available in stores. Cookies may be made out of hemp seeds. Try replacing nuts with sunflower seeds and pine nuts if you have any allergies to nuts.

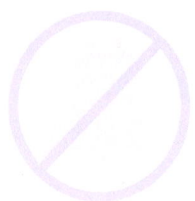

A NOTE ABOUT NUTS

The nuts I use are almonds, cashews, walnuts, pecans and macadamia nuts. You can use other nuts like Brazil nuts and hazelnuts. Many of the nuts can be substituted for each other to save you a trip to the shops. But there are a few unique properties of particular nuts that you will need to bear in mind.

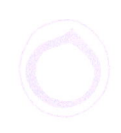

Macadamia nuts are very oily. The longer you blend them the more oil will be extracted. When I use macadamia nuts, I don't need to add oil. If you are going to substitute macadamias with almonds, you may need to add a tablespoon or two of oil to help the nuts bind with the other ingredients.

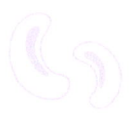

Cashews have a creamy texture when soaked and a very neutral taste. They form the bases of the cheesecakes and are used whenever I need the flavor of other ingredients to shine. It's easiest to plan ahead and soak the nuts overnight. If you forget, you can get away with soaking in warm water for an hour and blending them for longer. The creamy texture obtained by the cashews is only in part obtained via soaking. The rest of the work is done by a quality high powered food processor.

Walnuts and Pecans. These nuts can become bitter if they are old or you have purchased a cheap brand. Don't skimp on quality with the walnuts especially. Because these nuts have quite a strong distinctive flavor, they are perfect married with chocolate. I use them for chocolate brownies and bases.

Almonds are my 'go to' nut for many things because they are the least expensive and they are versatile. I use them to make almond milk and freeze the leftover pulp or dry it out so that it can be stored for later use.

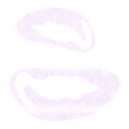

Treat **hazelnuts** like walnuts and pecans. **Brazil nuts** are a cross between almonds and cashews in their oiliness and creaminess. And if you have another favorite nut I haven't covered, please experiment with it. Just consider the nut's texture, oil content and flavor when substituting, and you should be fine.

VEGAN (NO ANIMAL PRODUCTS)

Egg-free. I don't have a problem with the humble egg but since these recipes are suitable for vegans and are also raw, I have omitted eggs. Eggs are used in desserts for thickening ice-creams and custards, they help bind cakes and cookies and they help things to rise. Instead, the raw food chef fills these needs by using agar-agar, chia seeds and psyllium.

DAIRY-FREE

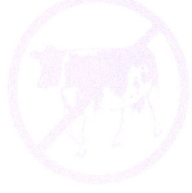

In almost all cases, dairy products in the form of milk, cream and cream cheese can be substituted in desserts. Use coconut cream in place of cows' cream, nut milks in place of regular cows' milk and cashews in place of cream cheese. These are the secret ingredients a raw food chef uses to recreate healthy versions of classic desserts.

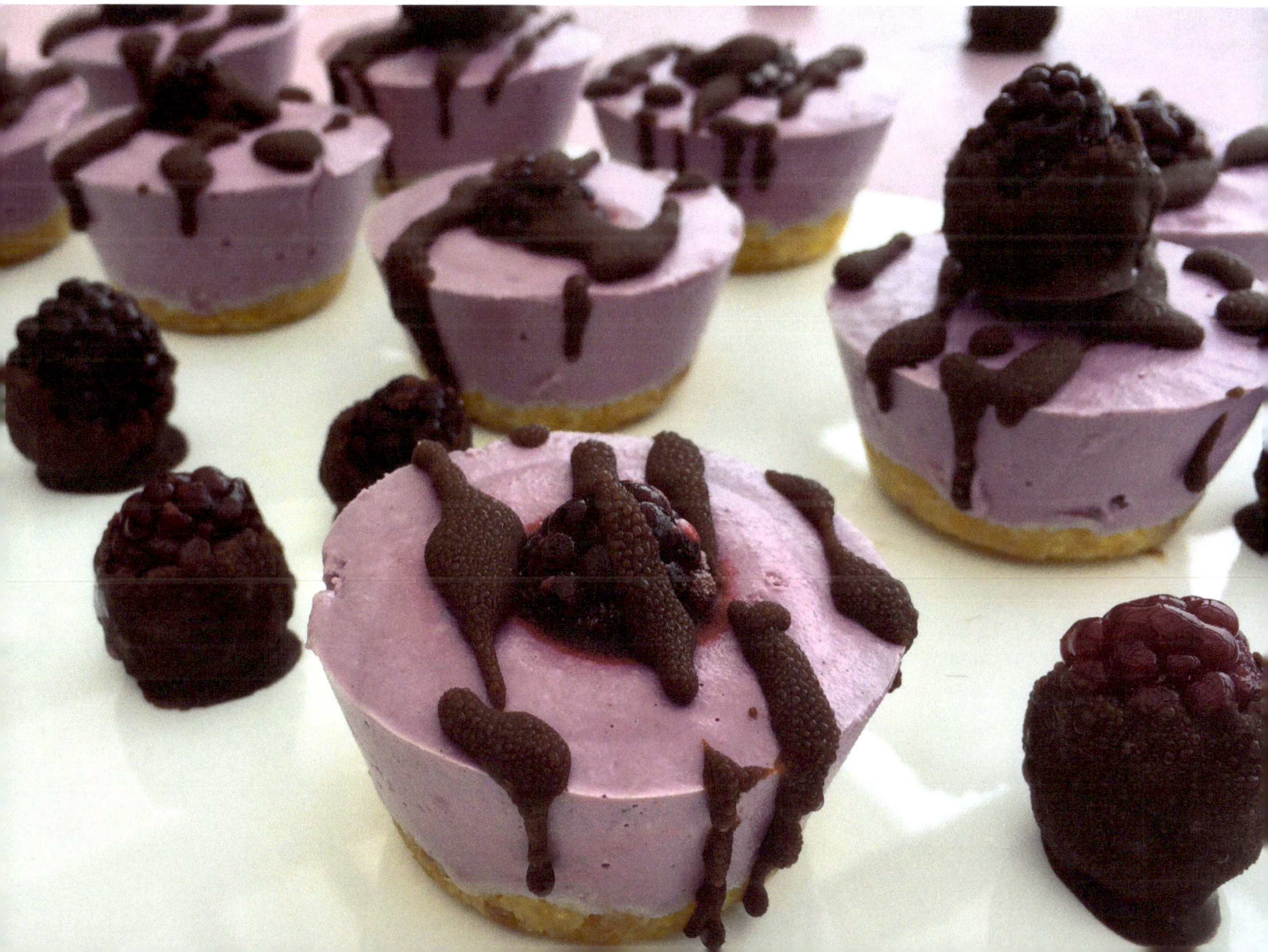

Almond Milk

WHY MAKE YOUR OWN ALMOND MILK?

Homemade almond milk is superior to any shop bought variation in both nutritional content and taste. But the real clincher for making your own is that the leftover almond pulp can be used in so many other recipes, from crackers, to desserts. After straining it into a nut bag or muslin cloth, squeeze the pulp to extract the remaining liquid. The pulp can be stored in the freezer in an airtight container for later use.

The Basic Recipe for Almond Milk

INGREDIENTS

- 1 cup almonds (best if pre-soaked for a few hours)
- 4 cups water
- 1 tsp vanilla paste
- 1 -2 tsp stevia or vanilla stevia drops to taste
- 1 tbs coconut oil (optional)

METHOD

Blend almonds and water in the blender for a few minutes. Allow the motor to run so that all almonds are pulverized. Rest a nut bag or muslin cloth inside another jug and strain the mix. Gently squeeze the bag to release all the milk. Pour the milk back into the blender and add the vanilla, oil and stevia. The milk can be stored in the fridge for a 2 - 3 days in a glass bottle or jug.

For a concentrated milk, repeat the above recipe but with only 2 cups of water.

Use up your leftover pulp from making almond milk. Dry it and store it in containers of one cup batches for ease of measuring.

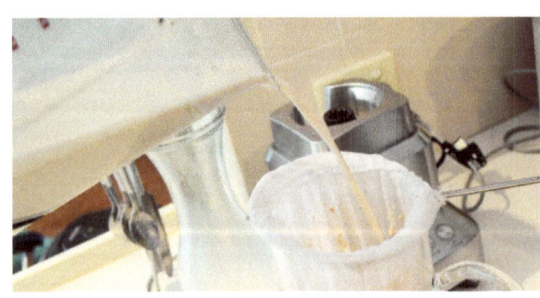

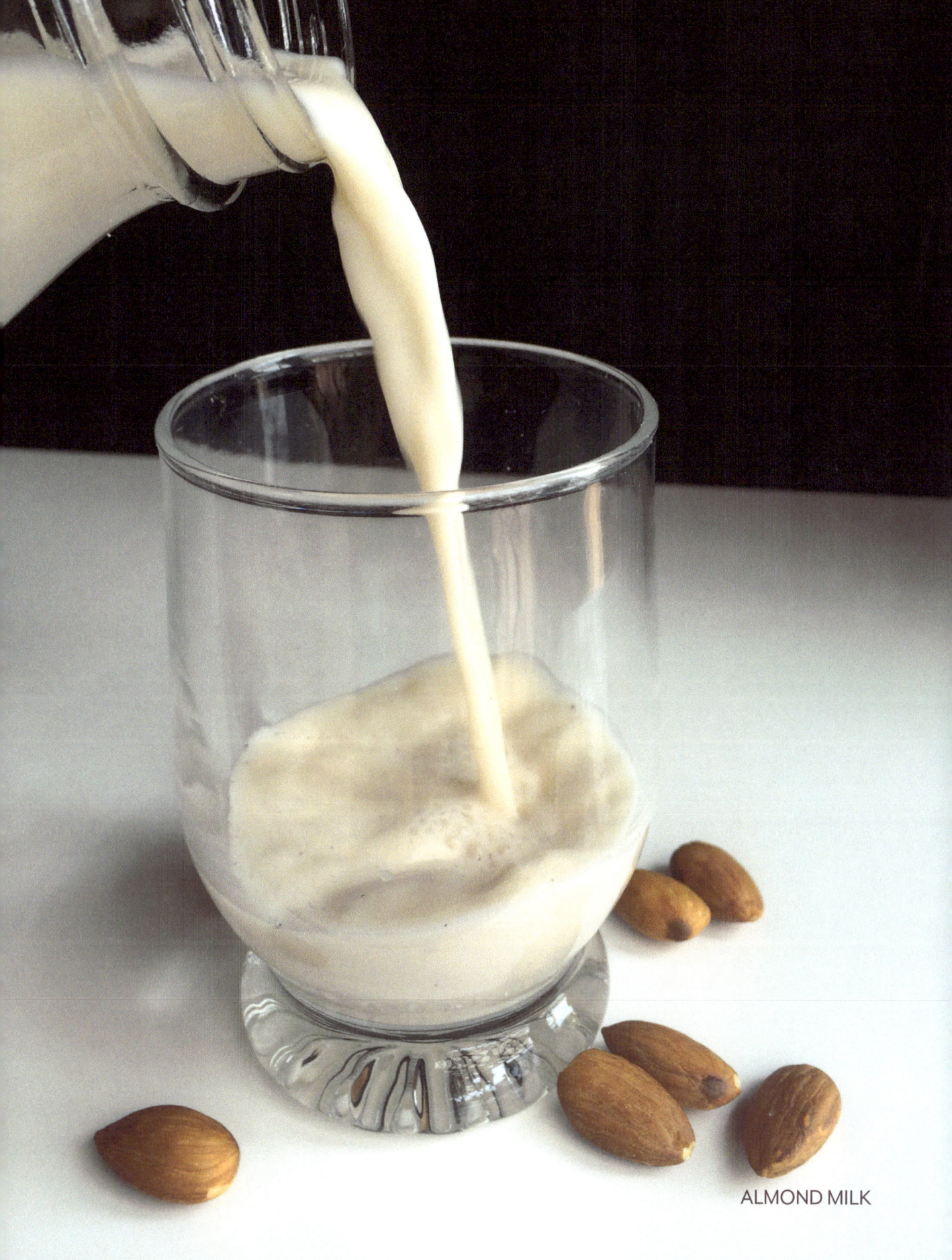
ALMOND MILK

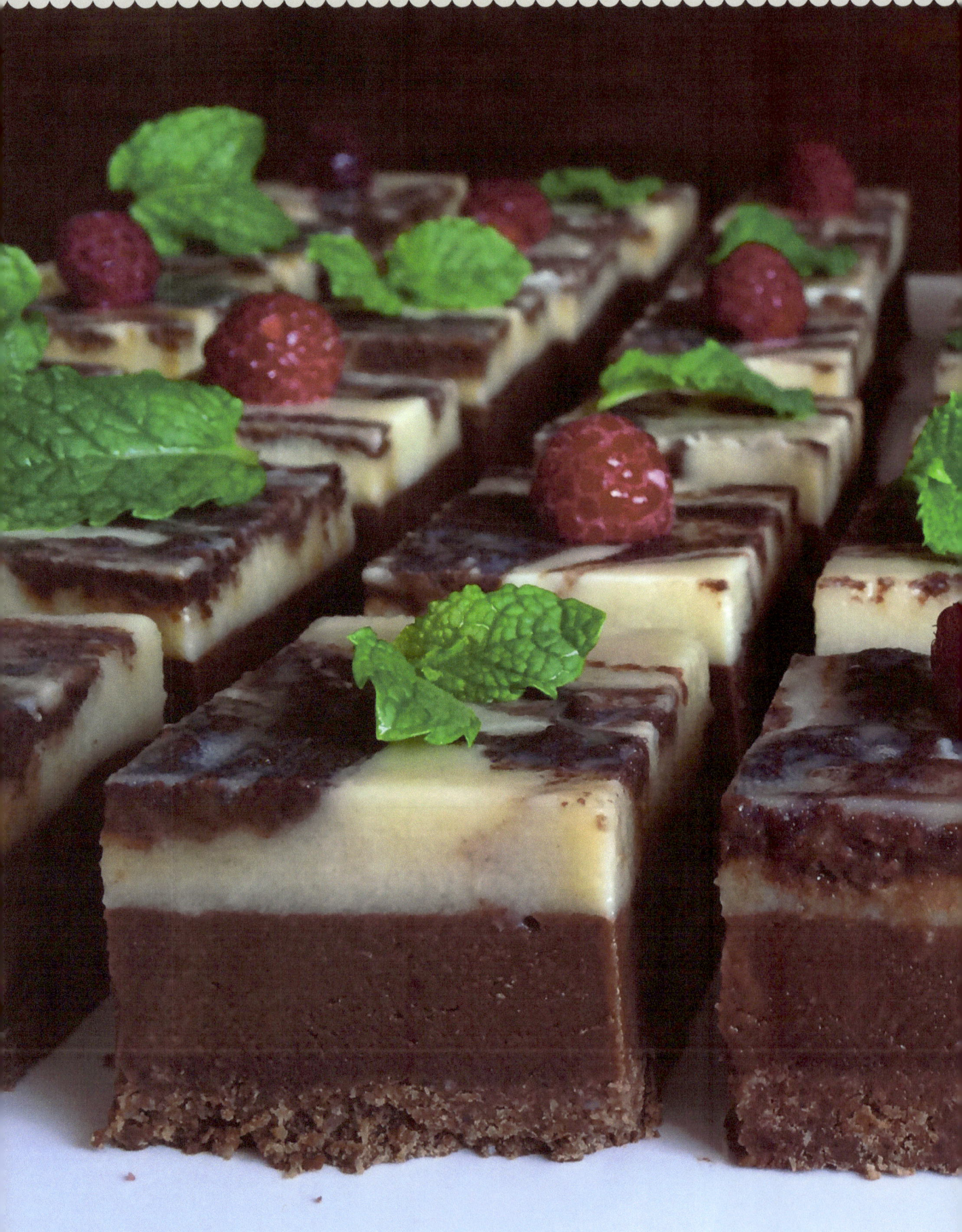

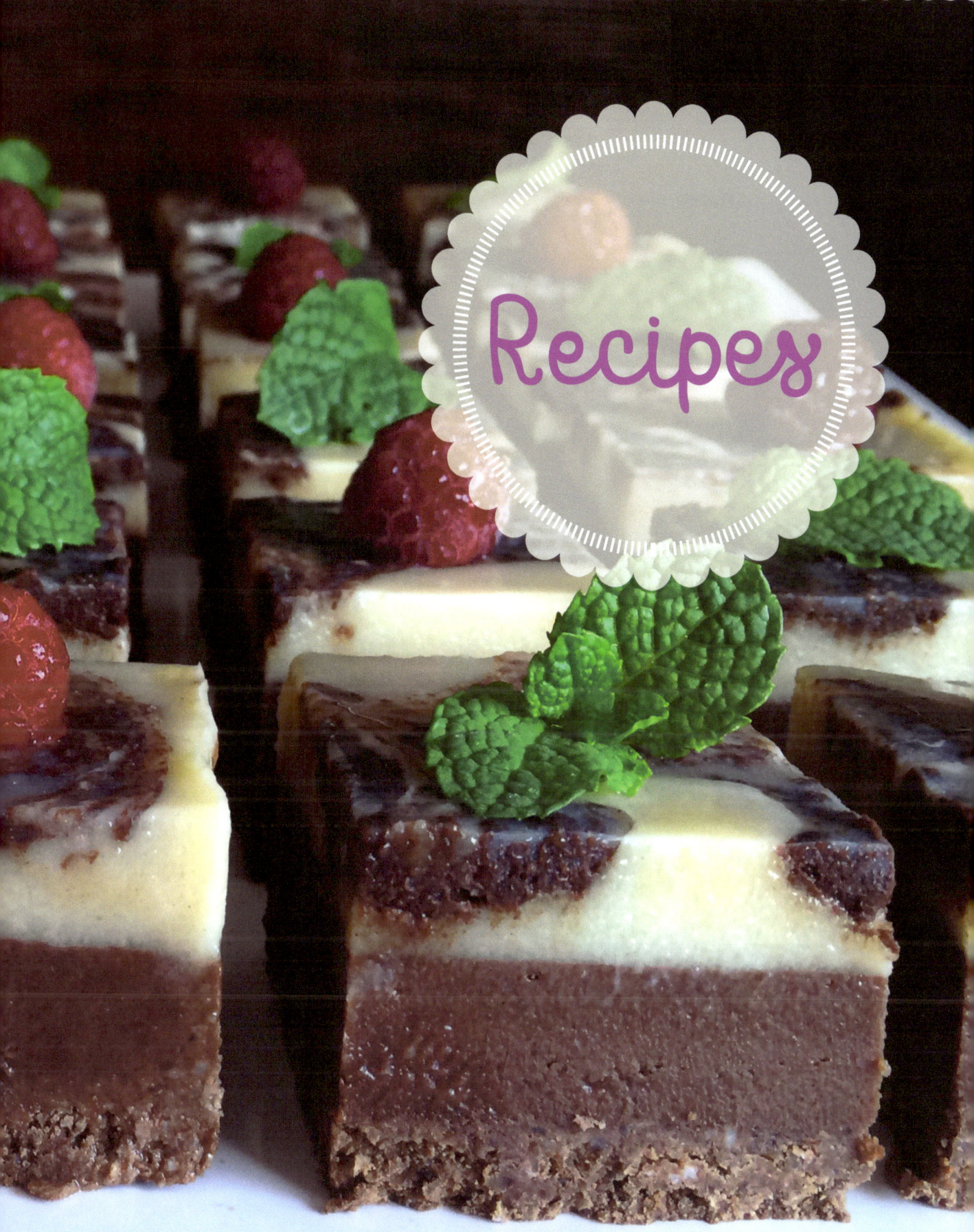

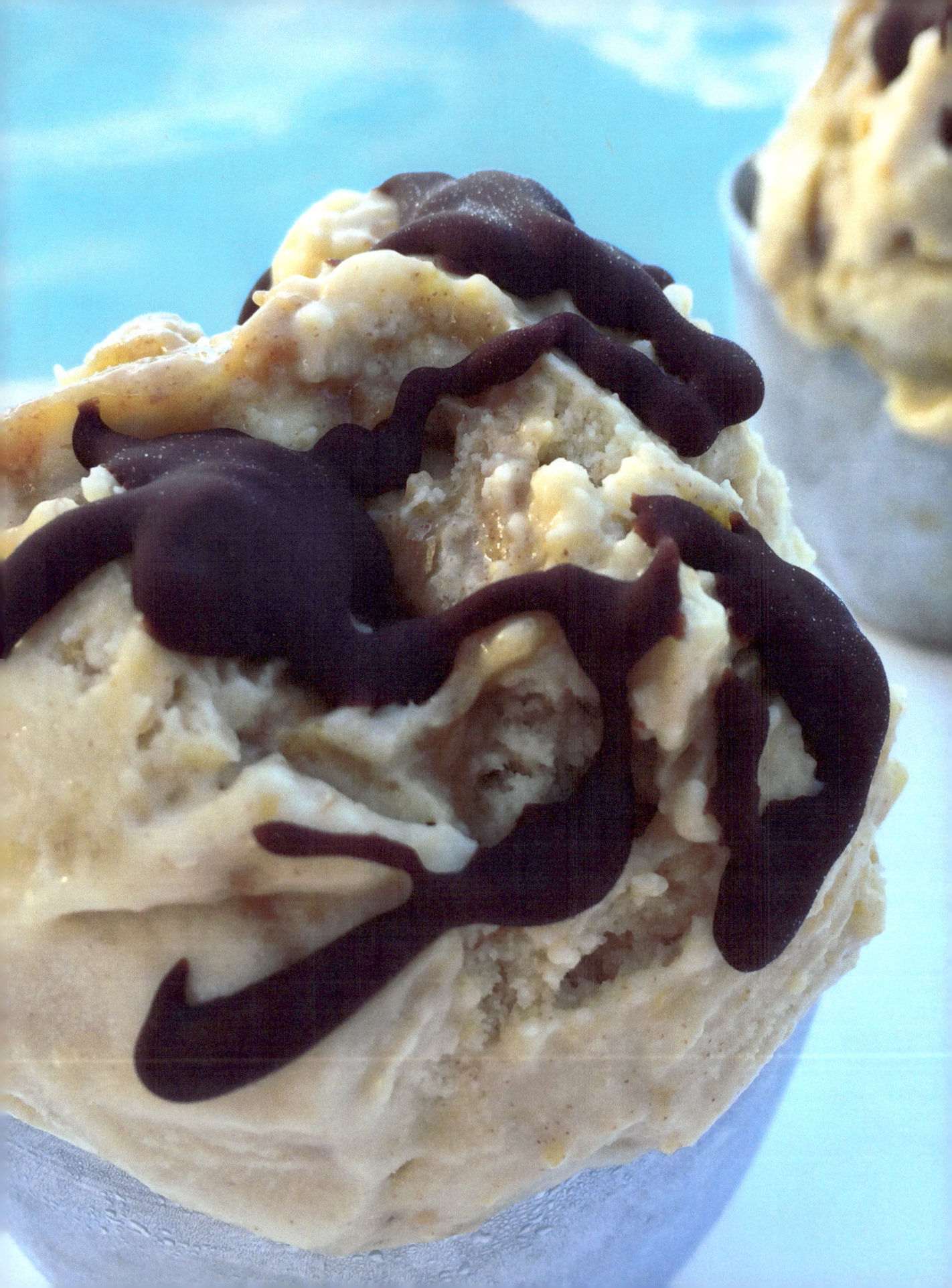

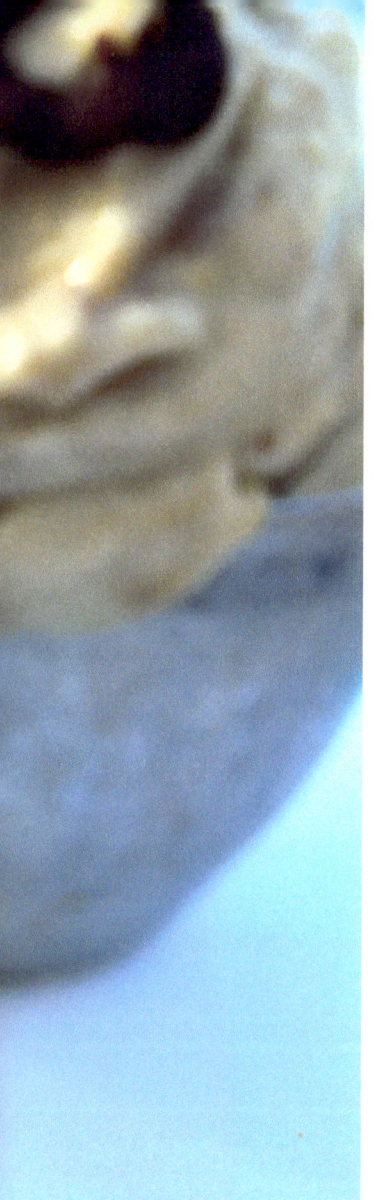

Ice-Creams

Traditionally, homemade ice-creams are a frozen custard made from milk, cream, egg yolks, sugar and flavorings. I've reinvented this summertime treat to healthy raw vegan standard, with resulting ice-creams that are excellent, from simple after-school snacks on a stick to richly decadent ice-creams worthy of gracing the table as the grand finale of a dinner party.

Ideally the unfrozen mix should be a little sweeter than you think optimal, as freezing reduces the sweetness. Using stevia is a way to keep the calories down. The recipes are not made from stevia as it has its own unique flavor which can leave an aftertaste if used in large quantities. It's used only as a sweetness booster.

An ice-cream machine is not necessary to make beautiful ice confections, but it does help. An ice-cream machine simultaneously freezes and churns. This breaks up the ice crystals as the ice-cream solidifies, resulting in a creamy texture. You can do this step by hand if you pour your mix into a bowl and then pull it out of the freezer every few hours to beat by hand. Alternatively, you can pour your mix into ice-cream molds. These can be purpose built, silicon cupcake molds or even ice cube trays work well. Have a look around your Tupperware cupboard, and you may be able to repurpose some old forgotten containers.

Strawberry Ice-creams

Although I admire it and try to emulate it, I'm not the world's most patient person. I get frustrated when the ice-creams don't come out of those ice-block molds easily. On a hot day, they start to melt before I've handed them out. My solution? Use silicon cupcake molds. So easy. Just peel back the silicon and they pop right out.

INGREDIENTS

- 500g fresh strawberries
- 270mls pure coconut cream
- 3/4 cup rice malt syrup
- 1 tbs vanilla essence
- wooden Paddle Pop (ice-cream) sticks

METHOD

Blend all ingredients in blender until smooth. Pour into silicon cupcake molds. Insert half a Paddle Pop stick. Snap these sticks in half by placing on the edge of the bench and karate chopping their length in half. Freeze until hard.

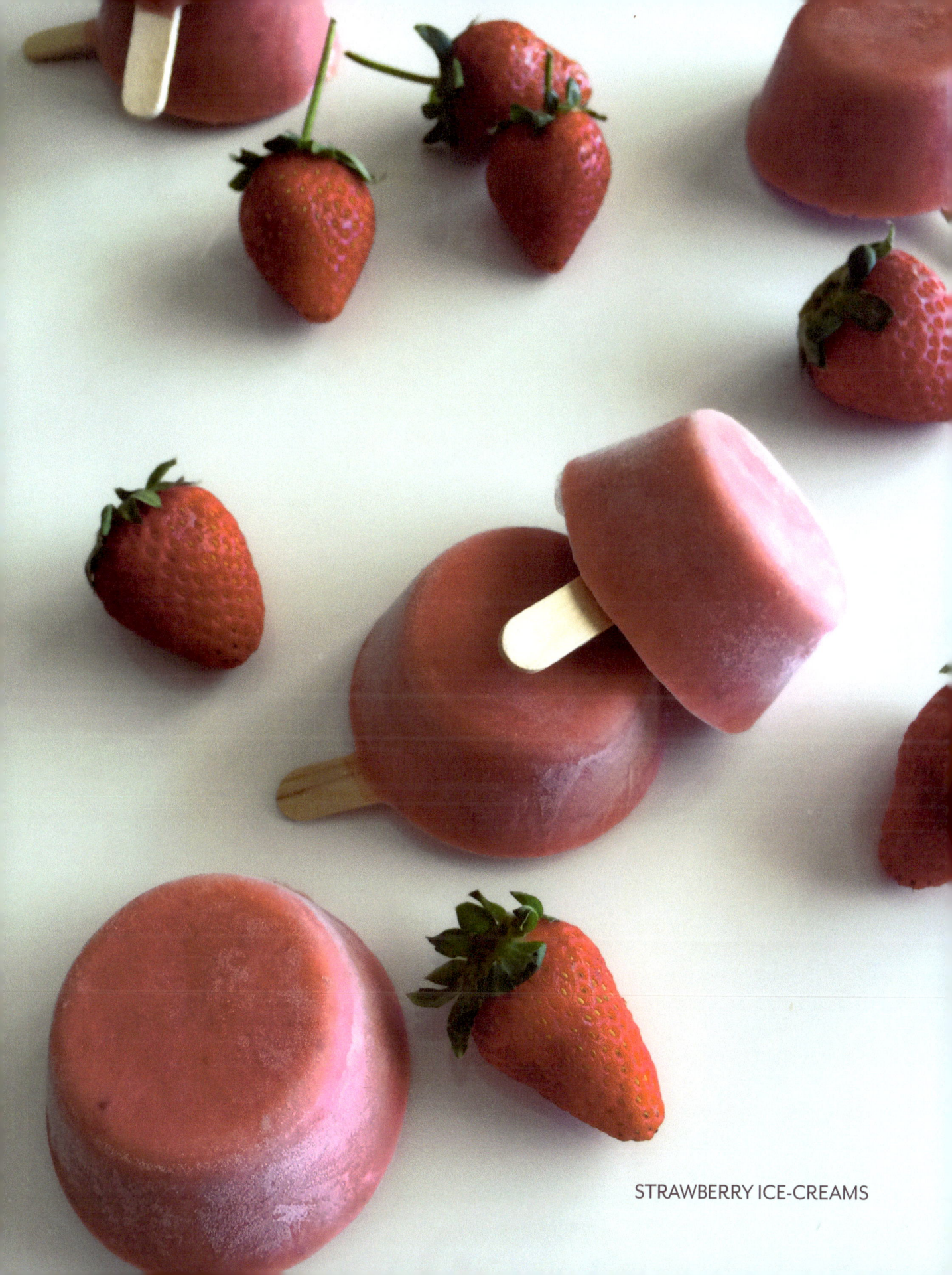
STRAWBERRY ICE-CREAMS

Raspberry Coconut Ice-cream Blocks

Messy faces, swirls of red and pink, lip licking goodness. Suck on these iceblocks poolside on a hot day for instant clean up. Don't you just love summer?

INGREDIENTS

Raspberry layer

- 1 cup raspberries
- 1/2 cup rice malt syrup
- 1/4 cup water (enough to get it moving in the blender)
- vanilla stevia drops to taste

Vanilla layer

- 1 cup coconut cream
- 1 cup concentrated almond milk (see recipe on page 14)
- 1 banana
- 1tsp vanilla essence

METHOD

Blend all the ingredients in the raspberry layer first and pour into molds, filling halfway. Freeze. Make the vanilla layer by blending all ingredients in a blender until smooth. Pour on top of raspberry ice-cream layer. For a more swirled effect, don't wait for it to freeze. If you want a clearly defined color line, then the first layer must be set hard to prevent mixing.

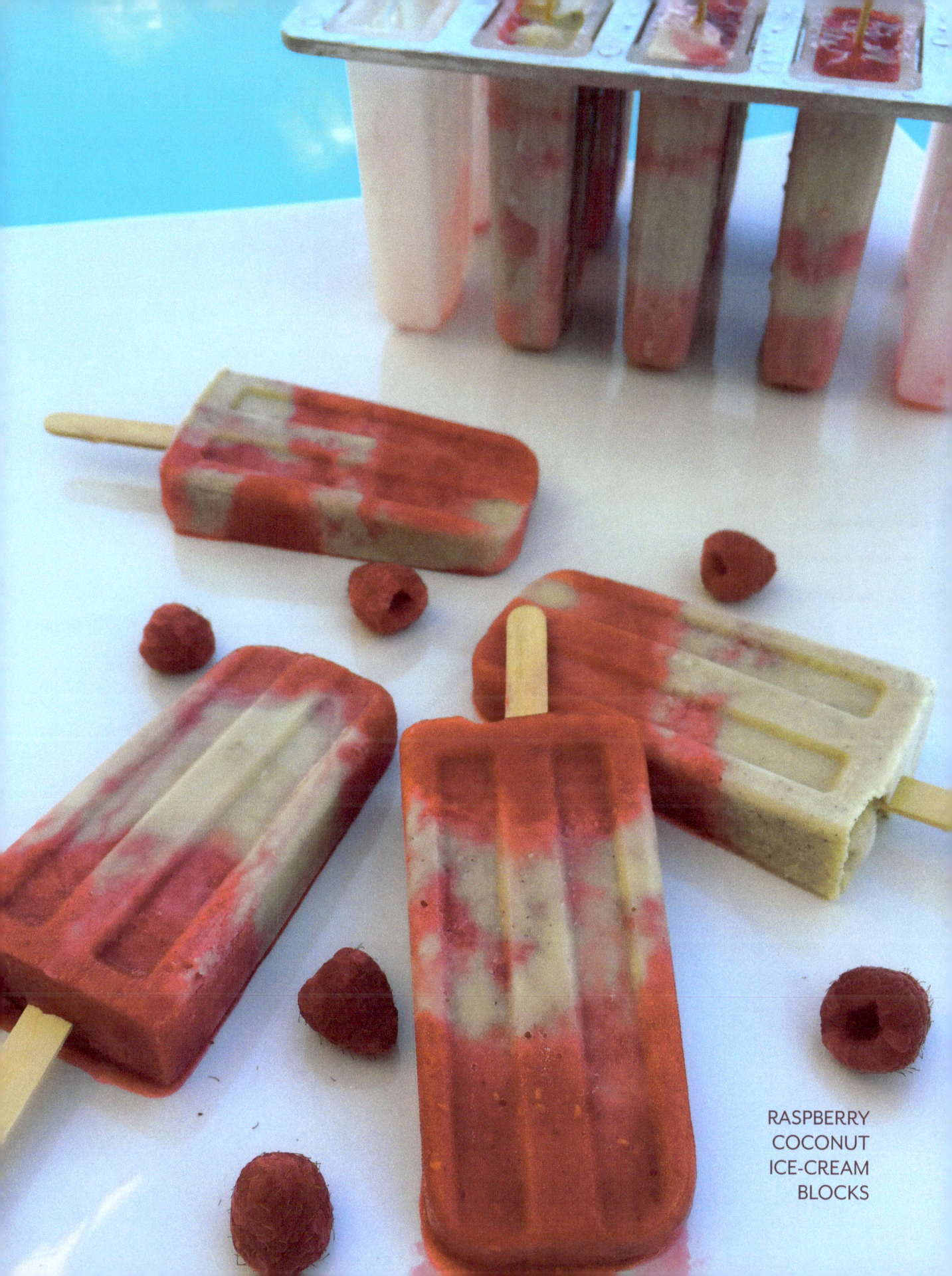

RASPBERRY COCONUT ICE-CREAM BLOCKS

Coconut Vanilla Banana Ice-creams

INGREDIENTS

- 2 cups coconut cream
- 1 cup coconut meat from a young Thai coconut
- 1 tbs vanilla bean paste
- 2 ripe bananas
- 1 cup rice malt syrup
- 2/3 cup cashews (soaked)
- stevia drops to taste

METHOD

Blend all ingredients in a blender until smooth. Taste. Add stevia drops if you need the mixture sweeter. Pour into ice-cream churner and churn for 30 minutes and then store the mixture in a lined bread tin in freezer. If you don't have an ice-cream machine, pour straight into ice-block molds.

SERVING SUGGESTION:

When frozen solid, dip blocks in chocolate or pour on chocolate sauce made from equal parts cacao powder, rice malt syrup and coconut oil.

Tip

Remember you want it to be a little sweeter than you think optimal as freezing reduces the sweetness.

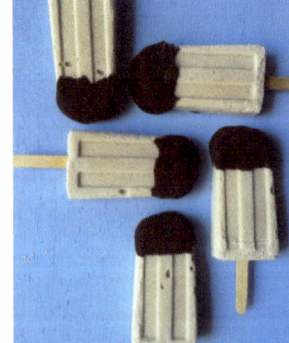
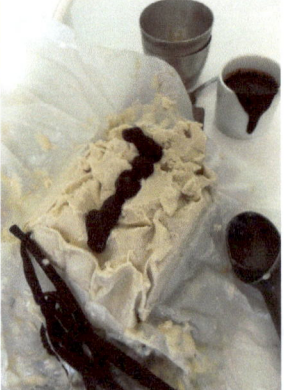

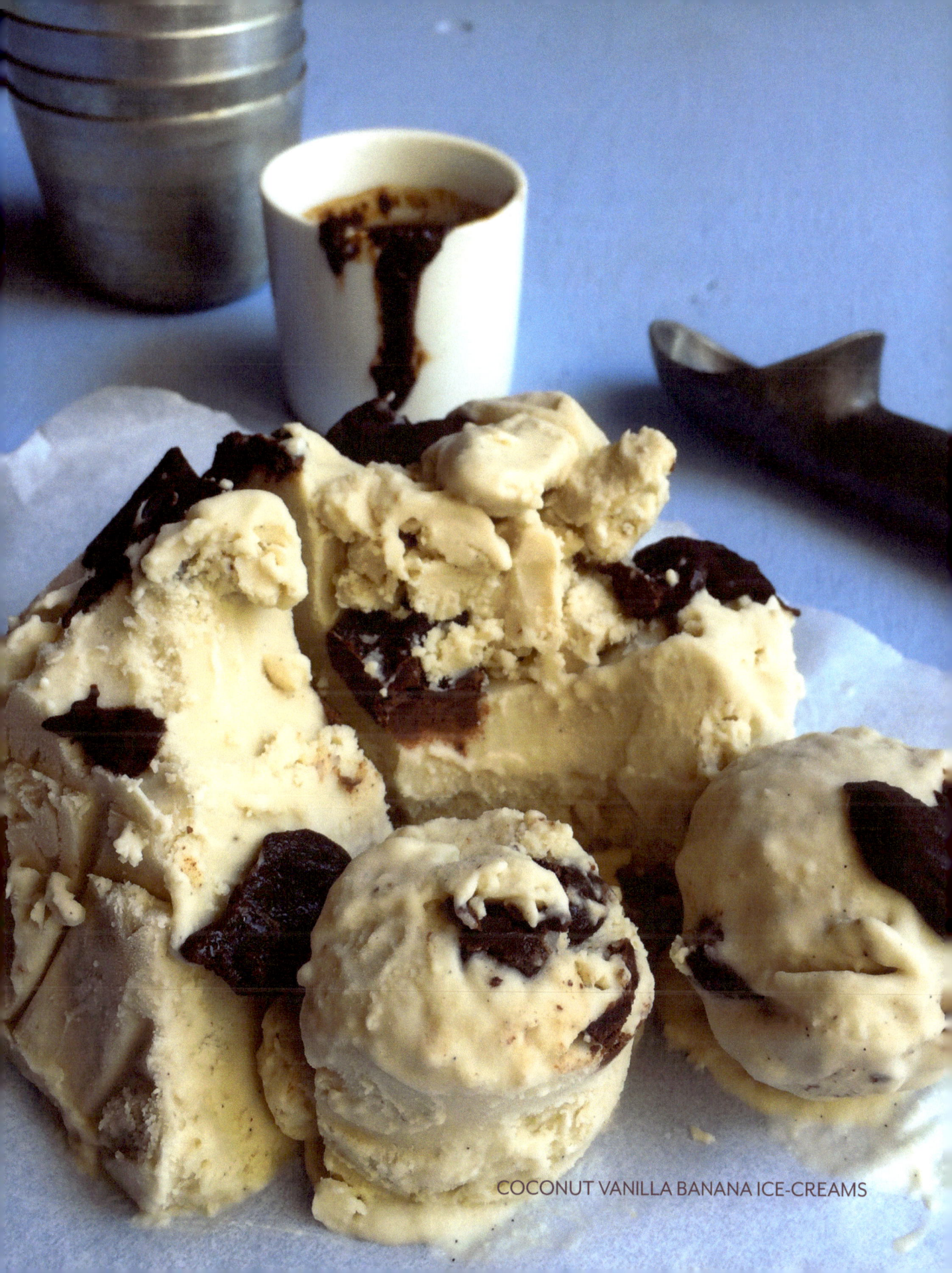

COCONUT VANILLA BANANA ICE-CREAMS

Mint Chocolate Ice-cream Blocks with Chlorella

I love being able to pimp my treats with green powders to achieve optimal health status. Chlorella is green algae that is effective at detoxifying the body cells. You can obtain it from a health food store. If you don't have it, you can make this recipe without it. However, it's a great superfood that is easily disguised by the mint in this tasty treat.

INGREDIENTS

- » 1/2 cup cacao butter
- » 1 cup homemade almond milk
- » 2 cups pure coconut cream
- » 1 large ripe banana
- » 1 1/2 cups rice malt syrup (or 1 cup rice malt syrup and then boost with stevia until sweet enough)
- » 1/3 cup cacao powder
- » 1/4 cup coconut oil
- » 2 tsp chlorella powder
- » 5 – 10 drops pure peppermint essence (food grade)
- » a handful of fresh mint (either for blending or garnishing)

METHOD

Warm the coconut cream and almond milk in a saucepan on a very low heat. Add all the ingredients (except the mint leaves, chlorella and banana) and stir until melted. The mixture needs to be body temperature warm only, so that the solids and liquids combine. Then pour the mix into a blender with the banana and mint and chlorella powder and blend until combined. Pour into an ice-cream maker to chill and churn. Then pour into a loaf tin to store in the freezer or eat immediately. If you don't have an ice-cream maker, then pour straight into ice block molds. Freeze for several hours until solid.

NOTE:

It's always easier to melt the coconut oil and cacao butter first over a bowl of hot water to measure it exactly, but if you trust your measuring skills you can measure then melt the fats in the warm almond milk and coconut cream.

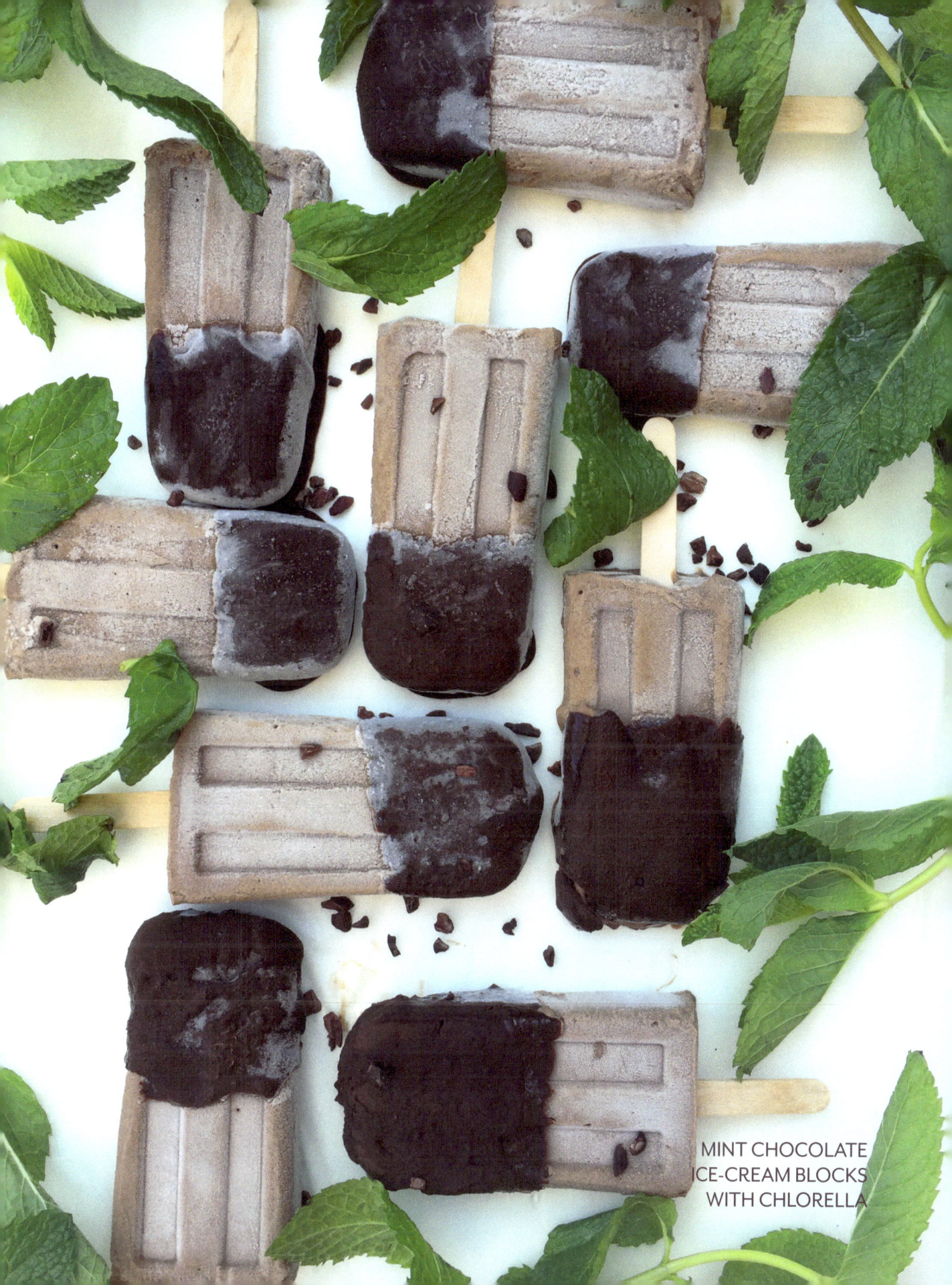

MINT CHOCOLATE
ICE-CREAM BLOCKS
WITH CHLORELLA

Mango and Coconut Yoghurt Ice-cream Bars

Whether you call them ice blocks, ice pops, icy poles, ice lollies or popsicles, these frozen ice-creamy treats are perfect for a hot summer's day and a great way to use up a surplus of sweet juicy mangoes.

INGREDIENTS

- 1 cup coconut yoghurt (or coconut cream)
- lemon zest
- vanilla essence
- 1/2 cup rice malt syrup
- 2 mangoes (2 1/2 cups)
- stevia drops

METHOD

Mix yoghurt, zest, and vanilla in a small jug. Purée mango in the food processor until smooth. You may want to add some stevia drops depending on the sweetness of your mangoes. Remember that when things are frozen they don't taste as sweet. Pour this mango mix evenly across the ten ice block molds and freeze. Continue layering the white yoghurt layer and mango layer. For a straight, clearly defined edge, freeze the ice blocks in between alternate layering. If you like a swirly effect, pour the layers on top of each other without freezing in between.

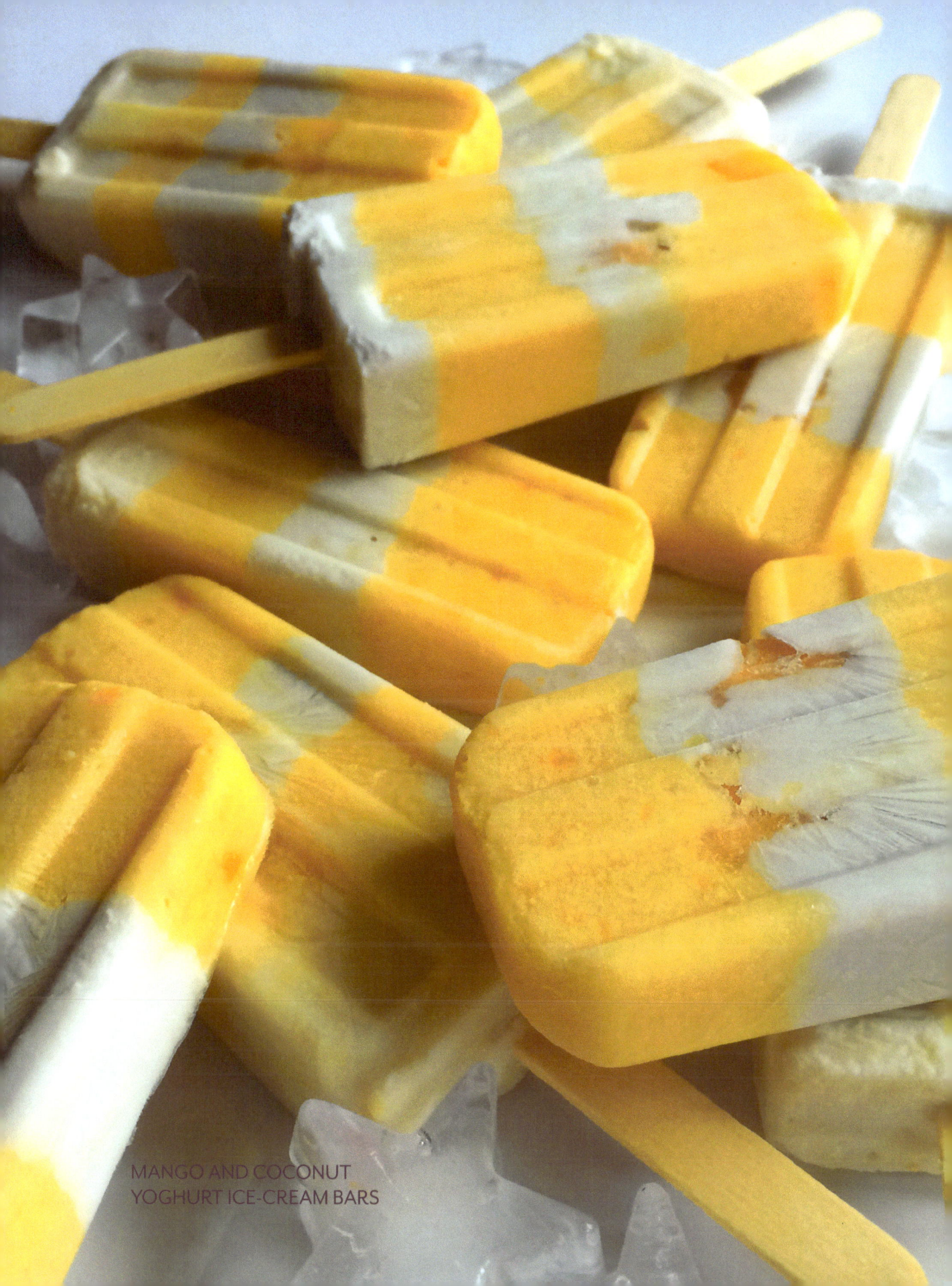

MANGO AND COCONUT
YOGHURT ICE-CREAM BARS

Coconut Mango Lime Ice-cream

INGREDIENTS

Ice-cream

- 800mls coconut cream
- zest of 1 lime
- 1/2 cup rice malt syrup
- 5 stevia drops
  (an easy way to adjust sweetness without more calories and without increasing the volume of ice-cream)
- 5 drops Doterra lime oil

Mango Purée

- 2 large mangoes (2 cups)
- 1/2 cup rice malt syrup
- Juice of 1 lime
- 5 Doterra lime drops
  (culinary grade essential oil)
- 5 stevia drops

METHOD

Ice-cream

Blend. Churn and freeze in ice-cream machine. Then make the mango purée.

Mango Purée

Blend until smooth. Fold the mango purée gently through the coconut ice cream and freeze several hours in a container lined with baking paper. To serve, dip your ice-cream scoop in hot water to create round scoops more easily.

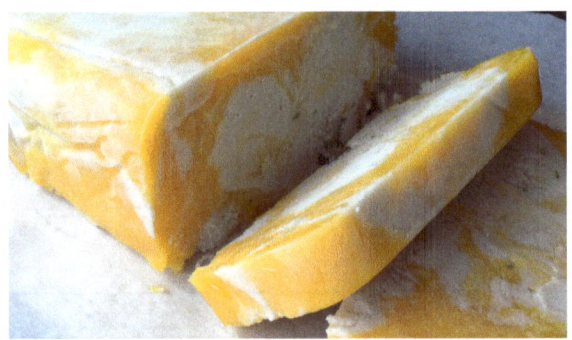

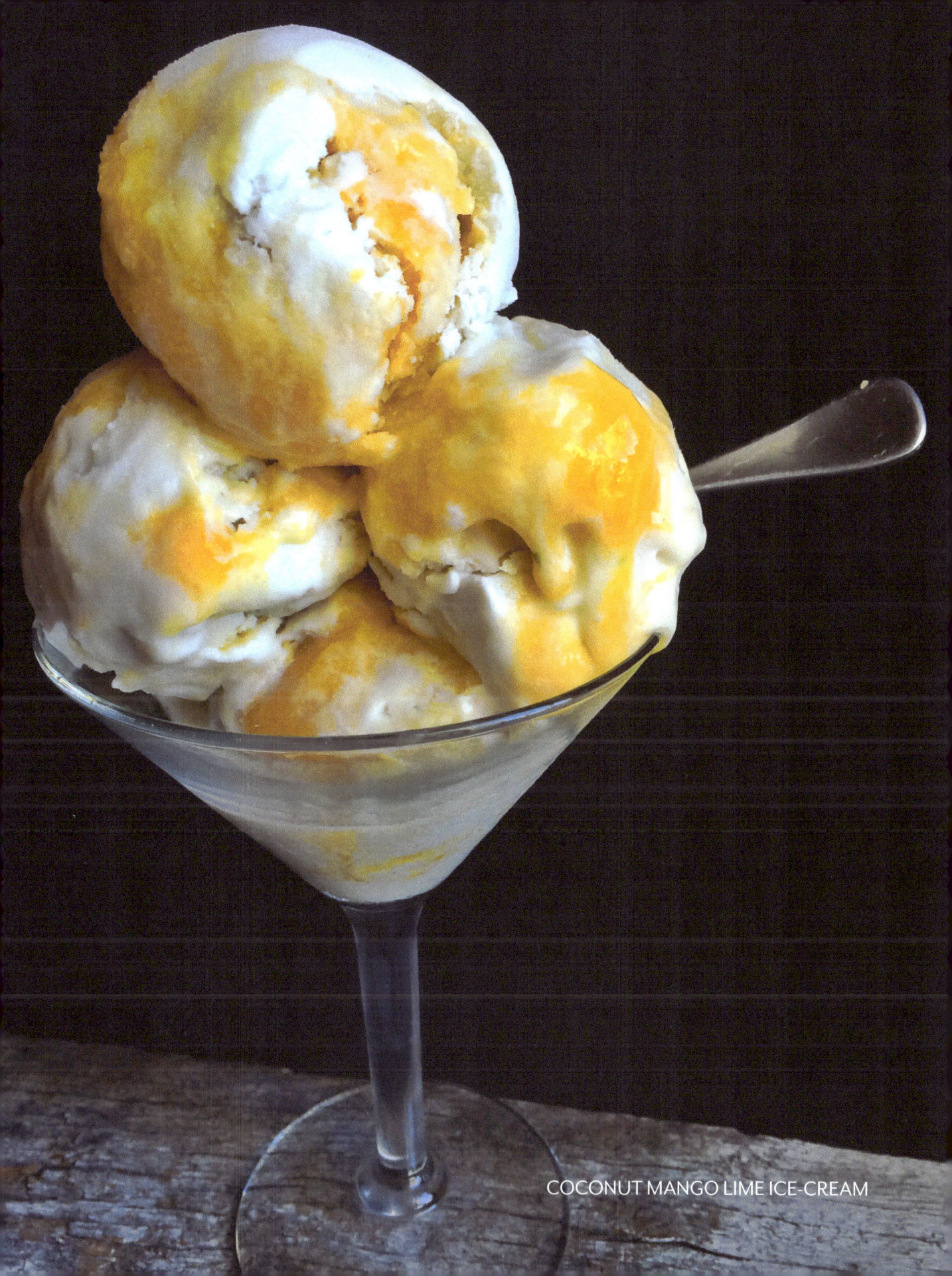

COCONUT MANGO LIME ICE-CREAM

Raspberry Tamarind Sorbet

Tamarind works well in a dressing but is also fantastic with fruit. This recipe started off as a way to use up some leftover coconut water. It turned into something so refreshing and delectable that it deserves its own spotlight. In fine dining restaurants it's customary to serve sorbet as a palate cleanser between meals. This sorbet is so delicious I'd just go ahead and have it for dessert.

INGREDIENTS

- 1 cup coconut water
- 1 cup raspberries
- 1/2 cup water
- 1/4 cup lemon juice
- 1/4 cup xylitol or other fructose-free sweetener
- 1 tsp tamarind paste

METHOD

Blend all ingredients in a blender until smooth. Pour into an ice-cream maker and churn until frozen.

NOTE:

If you use frozen raspberries this will be an instantaneous sorbet, ready to slurp and lick straight away, no freezing required. Store in freezer in a bread tin lined with baking paper.

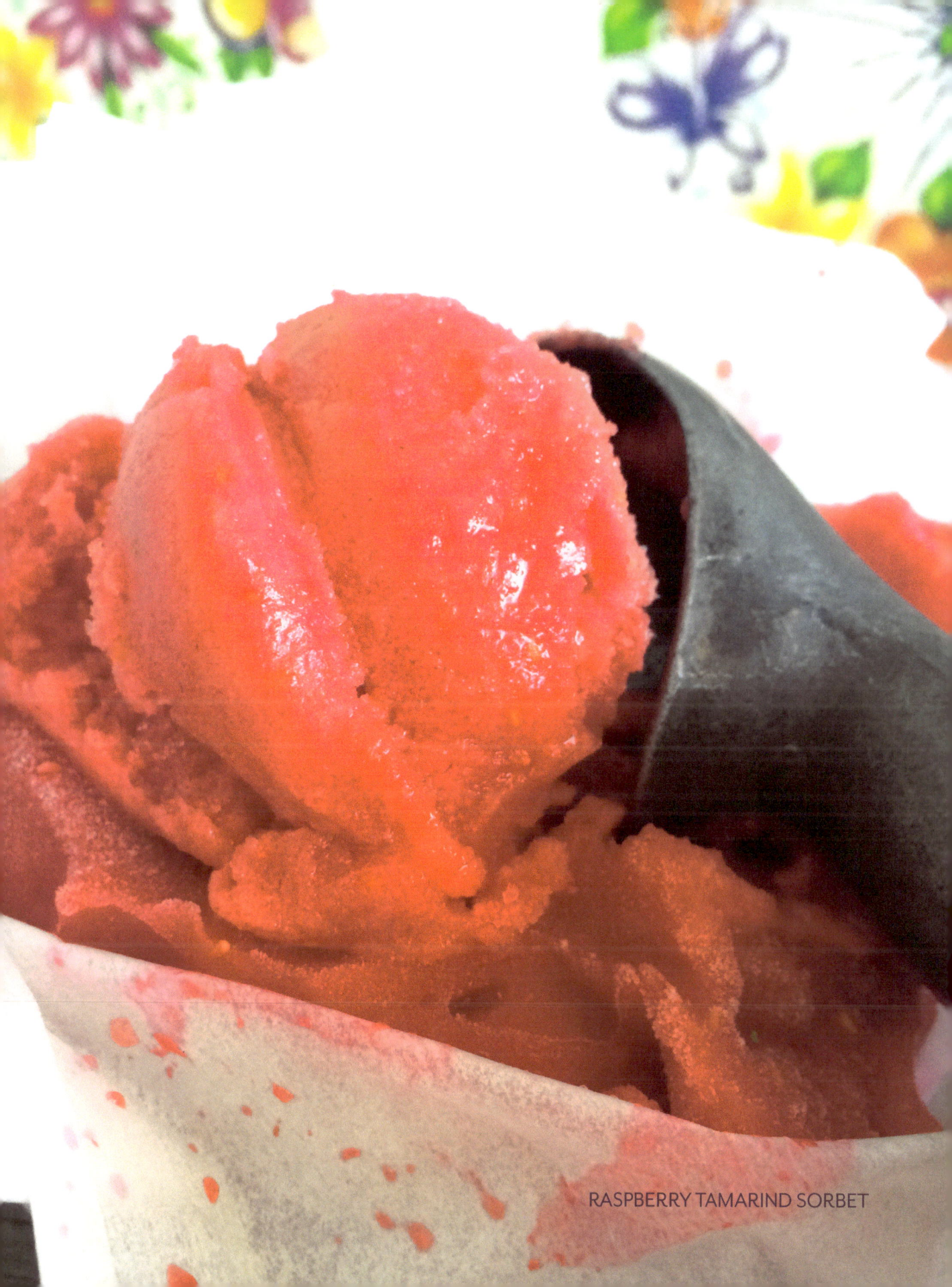

RASPBERRY TAMARIND SORBET

Chocolate Rosemary Ice-cream

If the thought of a traditional savory herb in a dessert sets you a little on edge, then you can leave out the rosemary. On the other hand, this might be the perfect opportunity to walk on the wild side and try something new. Go on, live a little.

INGREDIENTS

- 1/2 cup melted cacao butter
- 1 cup homemade almond milk
- 2 x (270mls) can coconut cream
- 1 large ripe banana
- 1 1/2 cups rice malt syrup
- 1/4 cup cacao powder
- 1/4 cup coconut oil
- 1 tbs vanilla essence
- 1 tbs rosemary leaves or 3 drops of rosemary essence essential oils (food grade)

NOTE:

It's always easier to melt the coconut oil and cacao butter first over a bowl of hot water to measure it exactly. However, if you trust your measuring skills, you can measure then melt the fats in the warm almond milk and coconut cream.

METHOD

Warm the coconut cream and almond milk in a saucepan on a very low heat. Add all the ingredients except the banana and stir until melted. The mixture needs to be body temperature warm only so that the solids and liquids combine. Then pour the mix into a blender with the banana and blend until frothy. Pour into an ice-cream maker to chill and churn. If you don't have one, then pour into cupcake molds for pre-sized ice-cream bites. This will make 1 1/2 liters of ice-cream, which means there is enough to fill the ice-cream machine and some left over to experiment with molds.

The purpose of the banana is to sweeten the mix so that less rice malt syrup is needed. This chocolate ice-cream tastes neither like coconut or banana because the potency of the chocolate and the rosemary overpower their flavors. This is a good thing. If you are not sure about rosemary in this ice-cream, then I urge you to go a little crazy. Experiment. Just add a drop at a time and taste. It does work.

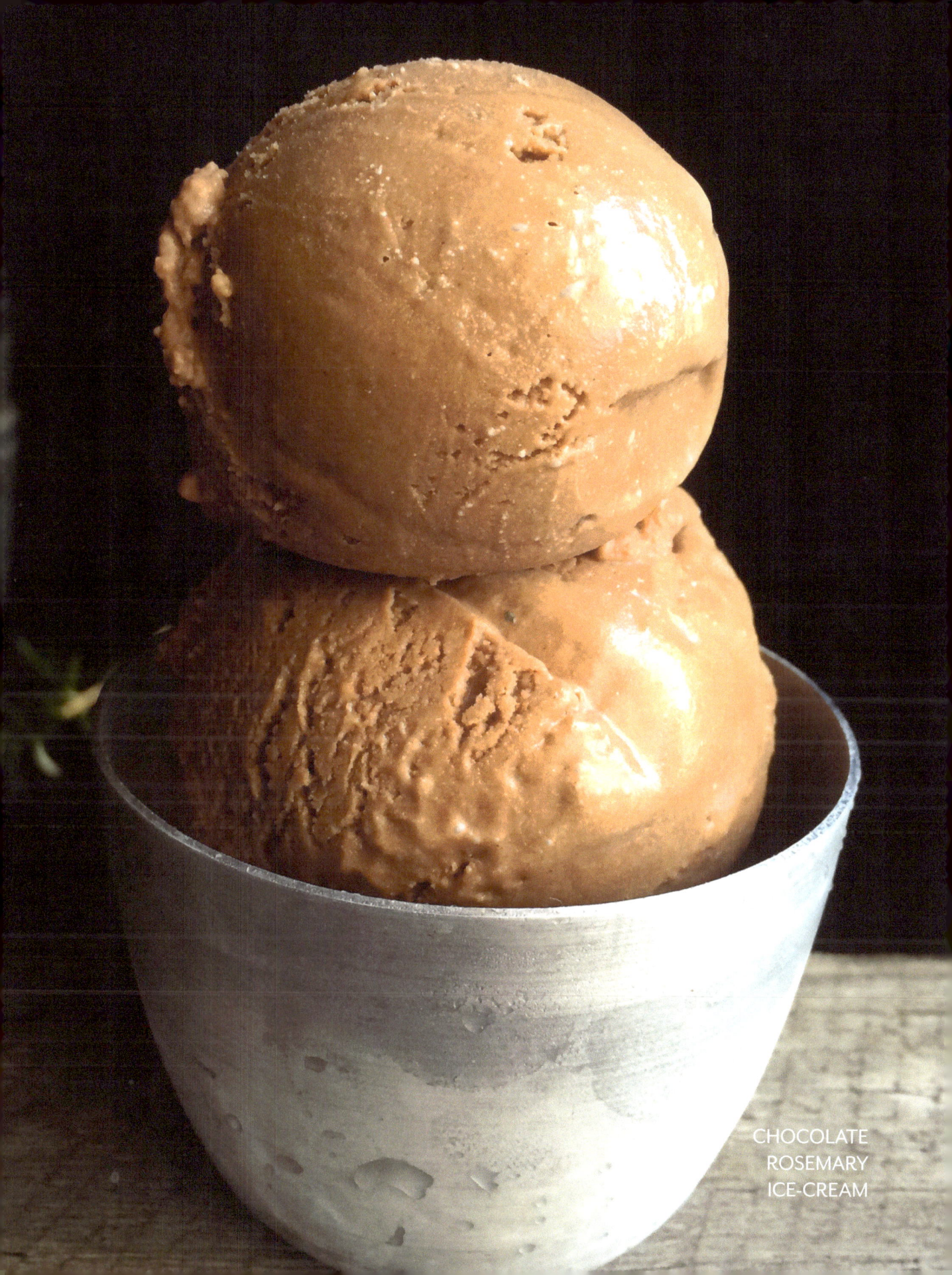

CHOCOLATE ROSEMARY ICE-CREAM

Lavender Blueberry Ice-cream

Simple steps and flavours that surprise are the marks of a good recipe. Trust me on this flavour combination. It is a bit weird at first, but everyone who eats it says the flavour gets more delicious with each spoonful.

INGREDIENTS

- 2 x 270 ml cans full fat coconut cream
- 1 cup (or 270ml) of home-made almond milk (just pour it into the empty can and swish)
- 1 1/2 cups rice malt syrup
- 1 heaped cup of blueberries
- 1 vanilla bean (ground in a spice grinder or scrape out the seeds if moist)
  or 1 tsp vanilla extract
  or 1 tbs vanilla essence
- 2 - 4 drops of food grade lavender essential oil

METHOD

Blend all ingredients except lavender for a few minutes in a blender until smooth and aerated. Add the lavender a drop at a time and taste in between until it's as you like. Pour into an ice cream machine and churn until frozen. Eat right away or scoop into a lined bread tin and freeze. Enjoy.

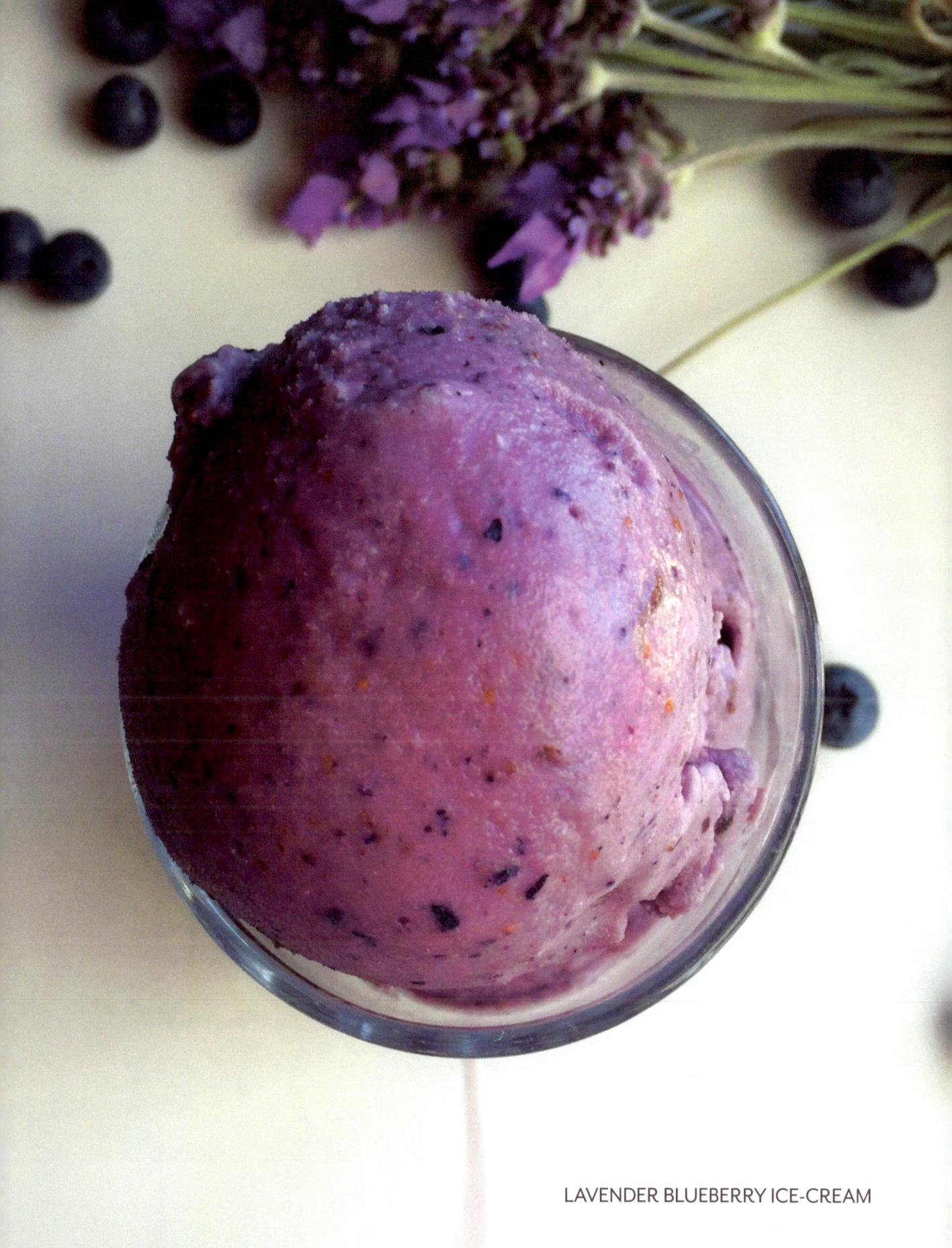

LAVENDER BLUEBERRY ICE-CREAM

Peanut Butter Cup Ice-cream

Life will never be the same again after you try this Reece inspired peanut butter ice-cream. Just as divine without the chocolate ripple. What are you waiting for?

INGREDIENTS

Ice-cream

- 400mls coconut cream
- 200mls almond milk
- 3/4 cup pure raw peanut butter (from health food store)
- 3/4 cup rice malt syrup
- 1 tsp pure vanilla extract

Peanut caramel ripple sauce

- 1/2 cup dates
- 1/4 cup maple syrup
- 1/4 cup raw peanut butter
- 3 tbs water
- pink salt to taste (1/4 tsp)

Chocolate sauce

- 1/8 cup (2tbs) cacao butter (could substitute with coconut oil)
- 1/8 cup cacao powder
- 1/8 cup maple syrup

METHOD

Ice-cream

Blend all ingredients in a blender until smooth. Pour into an ice-cream machine to freeze and churn. If you don't have an ice-cream machine, then pour into a container and freeze. Remove from freezer and stir every two hours to break up any ice crystals that may have formed. Make peanut caramel ripple sauce and chocolate sauce.

Peanut caramel ripple sauce

Blend all ingredients in a small food processor until a smooth paste forms.

Chocolate sauce

Melt the cacao butter or oil over a bowl of hot water. Stir in cacao powder and maple syrup until well combined. Once the ice-cream has frozen, stir through the caramel sauce so that caramel ripples form in the ice-cream. Don't over stir. Drizzle with chocolate sauce.

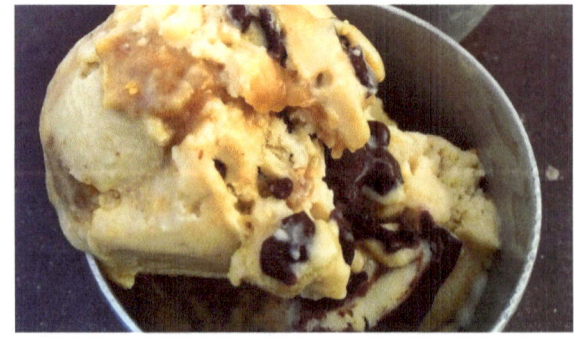

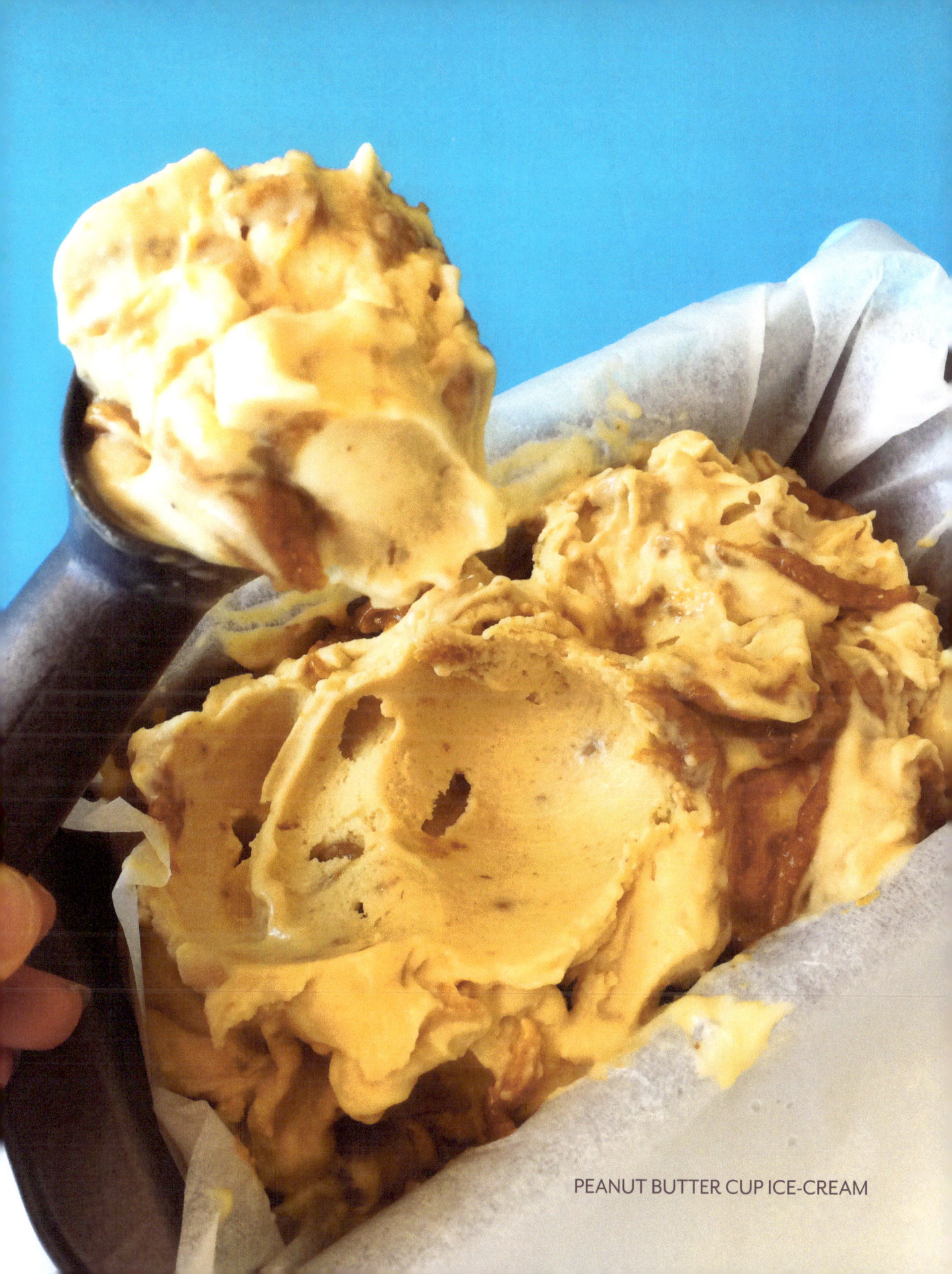

PEANUT BUTTER CUP ICE-CREAM

Brandy Black Forest Ice-creams

A Brandy Alexander cocktail is made of equal parts cream, brandy and crème de cacao. A black forest cake is a delicious chocolate layer cake filled with kirsch-soaked cherries and cream. I've decided to combine these flavors to make ice-cream cupcakes. Make 6 or double the recipe to make 12. They are stored in the freezer and perfect as a standby dessert for when unexpected guests drop by. I've decided to write this up as a 6 serving recipe just to keep the costs low for you. My regular recipe is double this amount. You could use traditional ice-pole molds but I always have trouble removing them so I thought I'd try the silicon since they make it a breeze to remove the frozen treats.

TO BEGIN:

Make a strong almond milk by blending 1/2 cup of soaked almonds with 1 cup of water. Strain into a nut bag and squeeze. Reserve almond pulp in the freezer for another recipe.

INGREDIENTS

Option 1 blend:

- » 1 cup coconut cream
- » 1 cup almond milk
- » 1/2 cup rice malt syrup
- » 1 tbs vanilla essence or 1tsp vanilla extract

Option 2 blend:

- » 1/2 heaped cup of fresh pitted cherries
- » 1/4 cup rice malt syrup or xylitol
- » 1/4 cup water

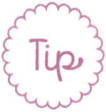

Tip: If you are using a 270ml can of coconut cream then just make up the difference with almond milk (230mls).

METHOD

Option 1:

Pour half of this mixture (1 1/4 cup) into a small jug and reserve it for the chocolate layer. Add 1-2 tbs brandy into the blender and mix. Pour into a large silicon muffin cake mold and freeze.

Place the reserved sweetened almond milk in the blender with 1 tbs of cacao powder. Taste and add more cacao if you like. Then pour this mix back into the little jug to refrigerate while you make the cherry layer. Wash blender jug.

Option 2:

If you decide to use frozen fruit, then I would recommend that you sweeten it with xylitol instead of rice malt syrup otherwise the syrup will freeze at the bottom of the blender and not mix. This won't happen with fresh cherries.

Pour this cherry layer on top of the semi-frozen brandy layer and then return to freezer. Wait until the top is set before pouring on the chocolate layer, then return to freezer to harden.

When ready to serve, simply peel back the silicon mold and pop each block out. You'll have raw vegan dairy free ice-cream that tastes so good even diehard naughty food fans will love this.

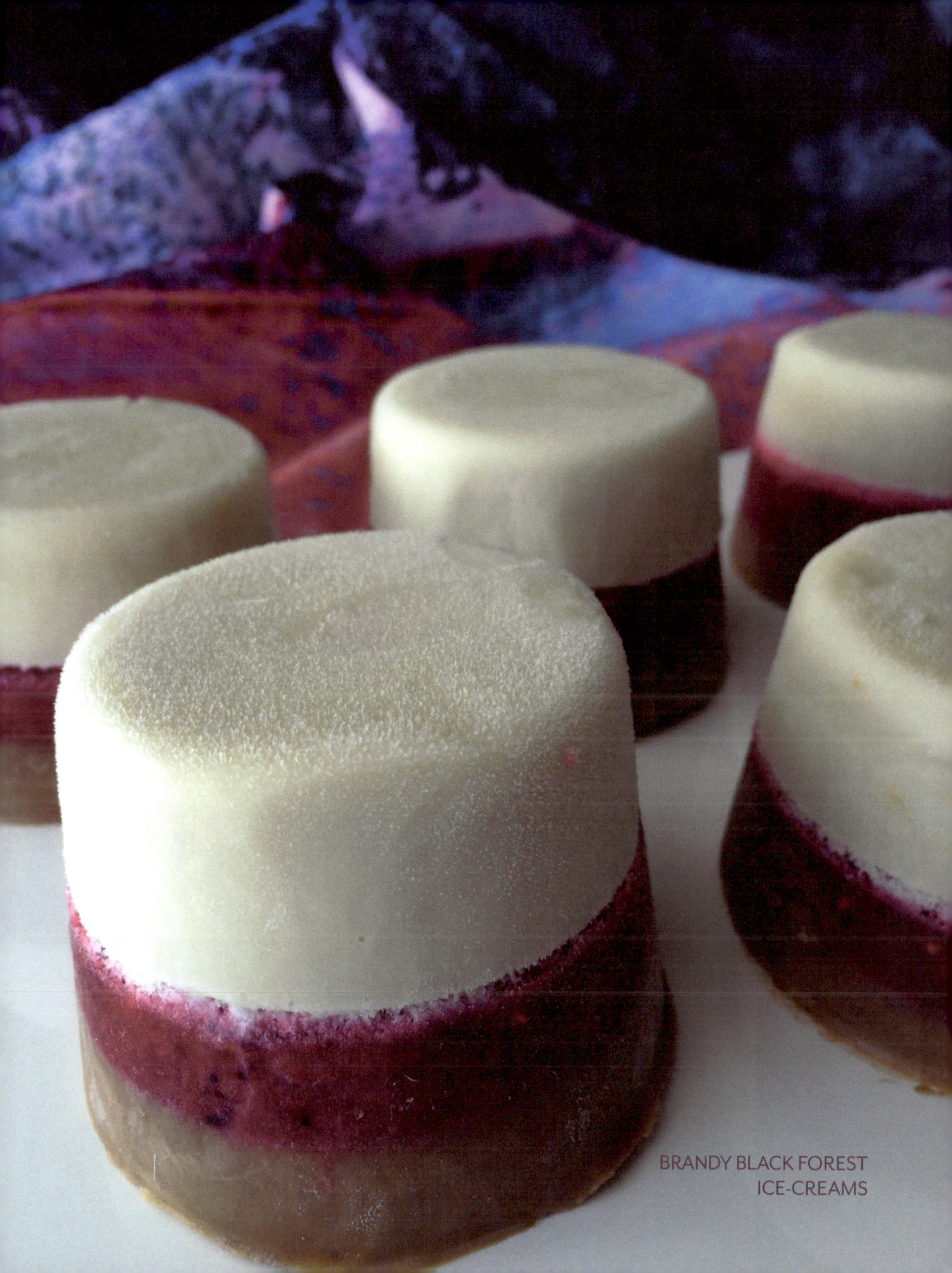
BRANDY BLACK FOREST ICE-CREAMS

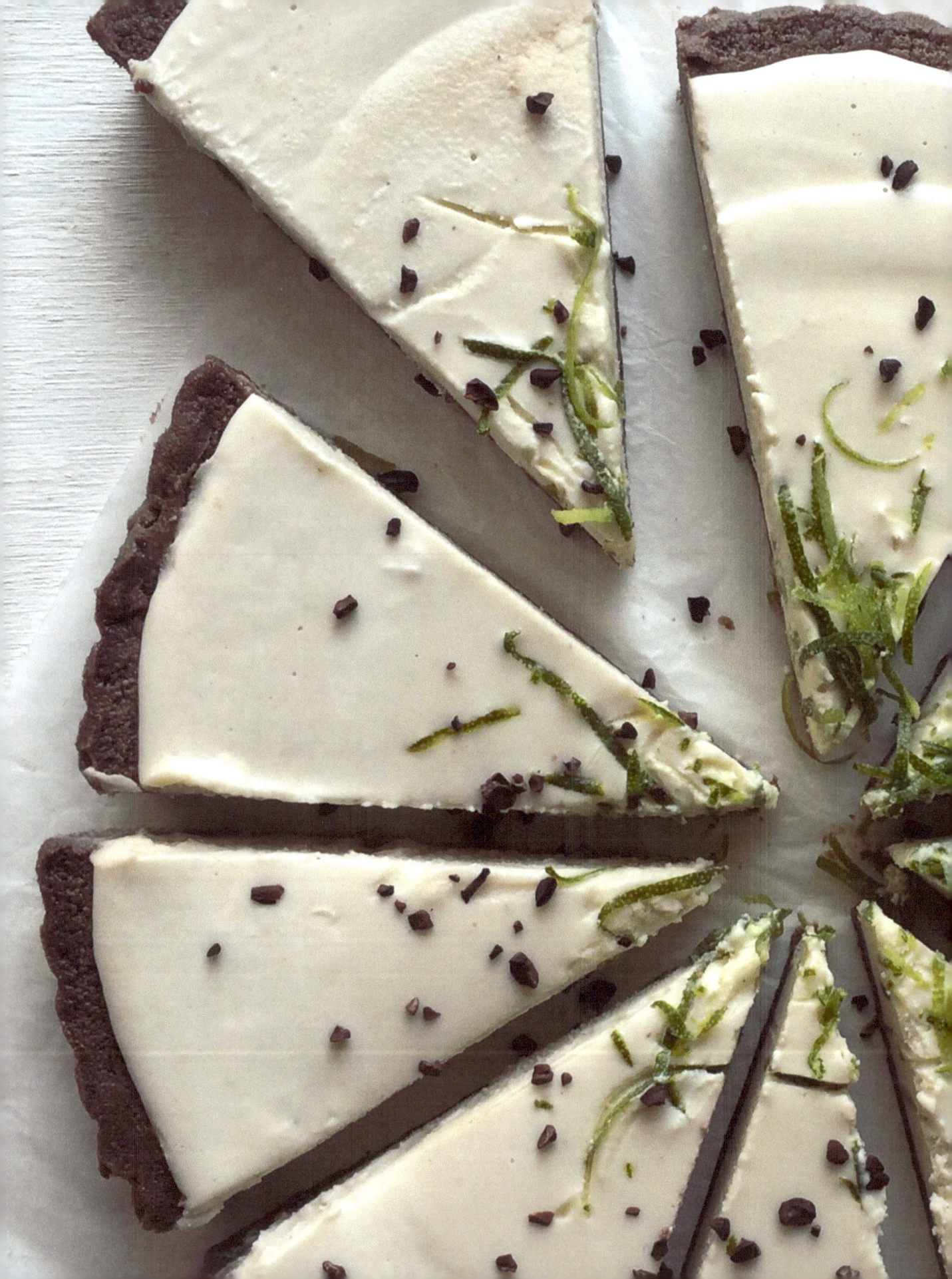

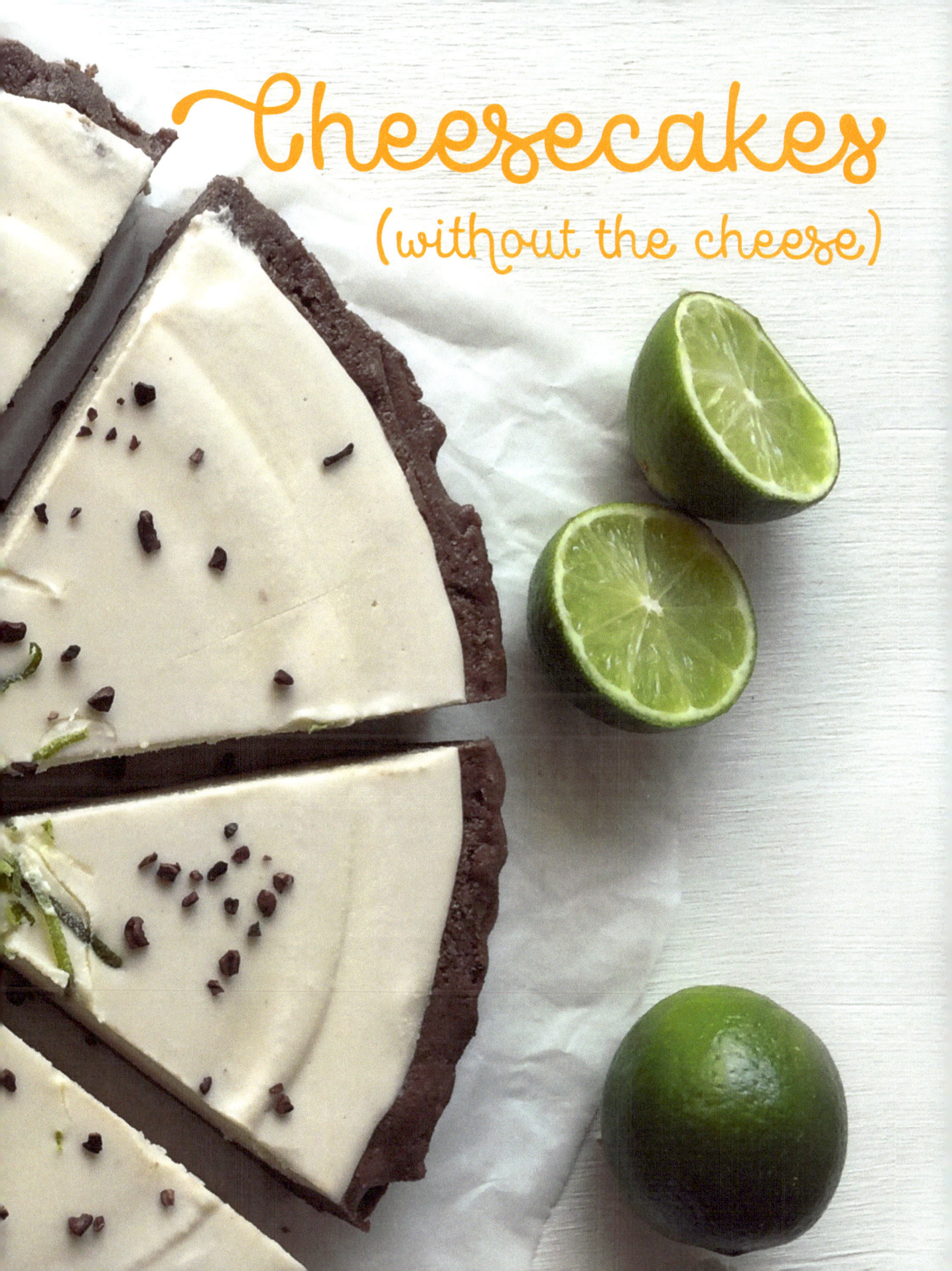

Cheesecakes
(without the cheese)

White Chocolate Cheesecake with Strawberries

INGREDIENTS

Base

- 2 cups almonds (pre-soak 20 minutes)
- 2 tbs cacao powder
- 1/4 cup coconut oil (melted)
- 1/2 cup rice malt syrup (add stevia drops to taste if you want it a little sweeter)
- pinch of pink salt

Cheesecake Filling

- 2 cups of cashews (measure then soak overnight)
- 1/2 cup coconut oil melted
- 1 tbs/30mls vanilla essence
- 10 white chocolate essence drops
- 1 1/2 cups of rice malt syrup
- 1/2 cup cacao butter melted (120g)
- pinch of pink salt
- 2 – 3 punnets of ripe strawberries (500g – 750g in total)

METHOD

Base

Blend nuts and cacao in a high-powered food processor. Drizzle in syrup and oil. Crackle the salt grinder. Once a dough has been formed, roll it into a ball and press down on a lined spring form baking tin. Smooth with a wet hand. Rest in freezer to harden. (The base, not you.)

Cheesecake Filling

Blend nuts and coconut oil until smooth and creamy. (Depending on your food processor this may take a few minutes. Don't rush it. The texture is key.) Add the vanilla essence and white chocolate essence to the melted cacao butter. Pour this into the food processor along with the rice malt syrup and continue processing. Add a pinch of salt to taste. Pour half the mixture on top of the base and return to freezer to set for an hour. Remove and place one punnet of sliced and hulled strawberries on top of the white chocolate cheesecake which is now set. Pour over the remaining cheesecake mixture and place in the fridge to harden. Once firm, top with the remaining strawberries.

NOTE

This is not a good recipe to store in the freezer as the strawberries will go rock hard. If you want to prepare this ahead of time, or to keep it for a few days in the fridge or freezer, make it without the strawberries in the middle and on top. When you are ready to serve, place generous amounts of strawberries on top. Don't skimp on the strawberries.

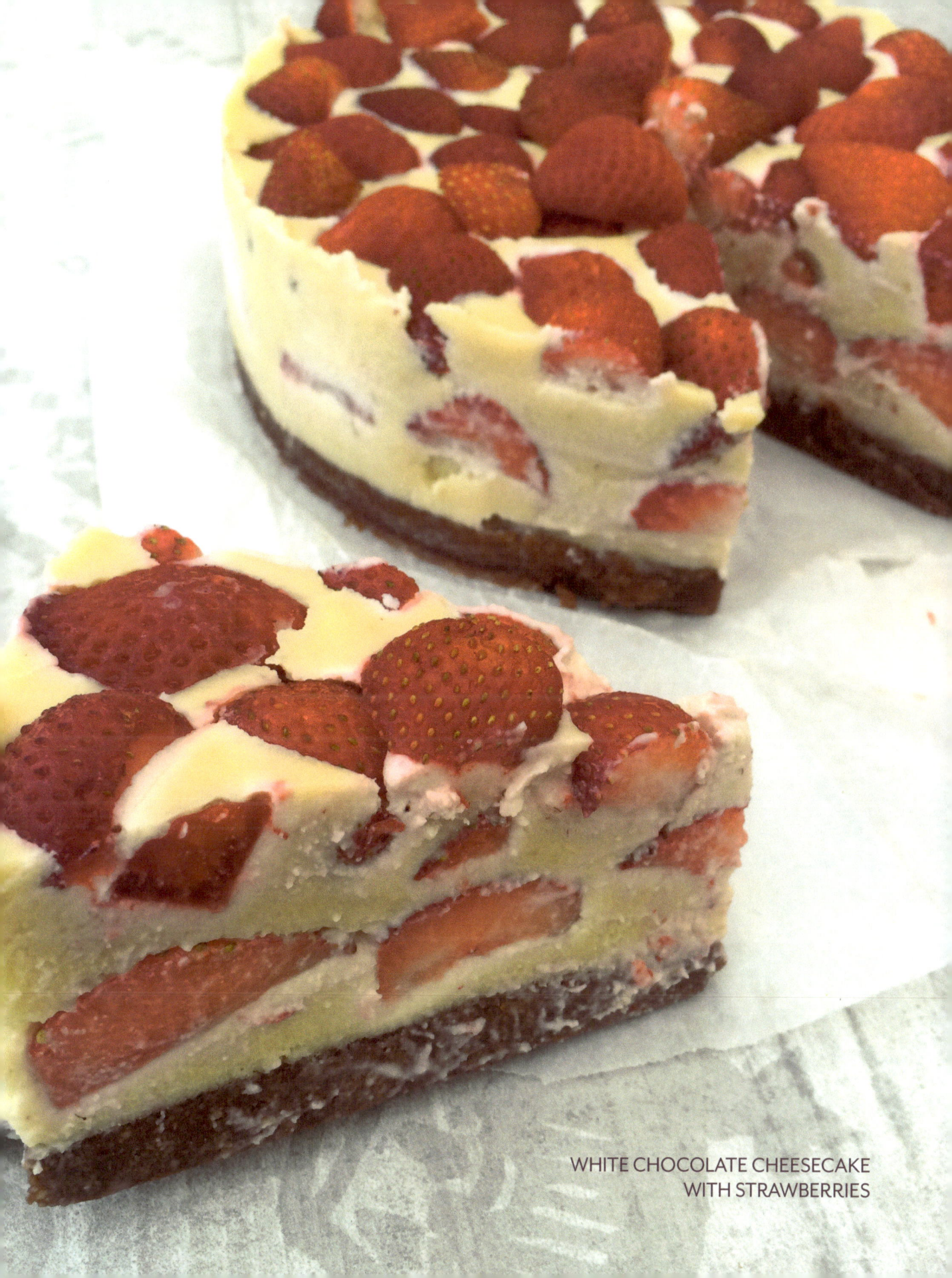

WHITE CHOCOLATE CHEESECAKE
WITH STRAWBERRIES

Banana Strawberry Layered Cheesecake

INGREDIENTS

Crust

- 1 1/2 cups almonds (can use the leftover pulp from almond milk)
- 1/2 cup desiccated coconut
- 1/4 cup coconut oil
- 1/4 cup rice malt syrup

Banana Passionfruit Layer

- 1 cup cashews (soaked overnight)
- 2 large ripe bananas
- 3/4 cup coconut cream
- 1/4 cup rice malt syrup
- 1/4 cup passionfruit pulp
- 1/4 cup coconut oil or coconut paste
- 1 tbs vanilla extract
- a grind of Himalayan salt

Strawberry Layer

- 1 cup cashews (soaked overnight)
- 250g punnet of strawberries
- 1/2 cup rice malt syrup
- 1/3 cup coconut oil
- 20 vanilla stevia drops or one eye dropper full
- extra strawberries to layer in between

Strawberry Coulis

- 1 x 250 g punnet of strawberries (minus the few used to scatter in the middle of the cheesecake layers)
- 2 tbs rice malt syrup or xylitol
- 1 – 2 passionfruit

METHOD

Crust

Blend all ingredients in a food processor, adding the oil last. Once a dough-like texture is reached, press into a lined spring form tin with the back of a spoon. Refrigerate.

Banana Passionfruit Layer

Blend cashew nuts until creamy, then add the rest of the ingredients into the food processor and continue blending until very smooth. Pour onto the base then return to freezer to set.

Strawberry Layer

Blend nuts in food processor until creamy then add remaining ingredients and continue blending until smooth. Remove cheesecake from freezer. Place some additional strawberry slices on top of the banana layer before pouring on the strawberry cheesecake layer. Take these from the punnet of strawberries used to make the coulis in the next step. Pour on strawberry layer. Return to freezer to set.

Strawberry Coulis

Blend all ingredients in the blender. Pour into a clean squeeze bottle to make a stripy effect on your cheesecake or just pour straight on top of the cheesecake. Allow a few hours for the mixture to set but not to freeze solid. This cheesecake can be stored in the freezer but is best eaten when it has warmed for half an hour at room temperature. Slice while semi-frozen.

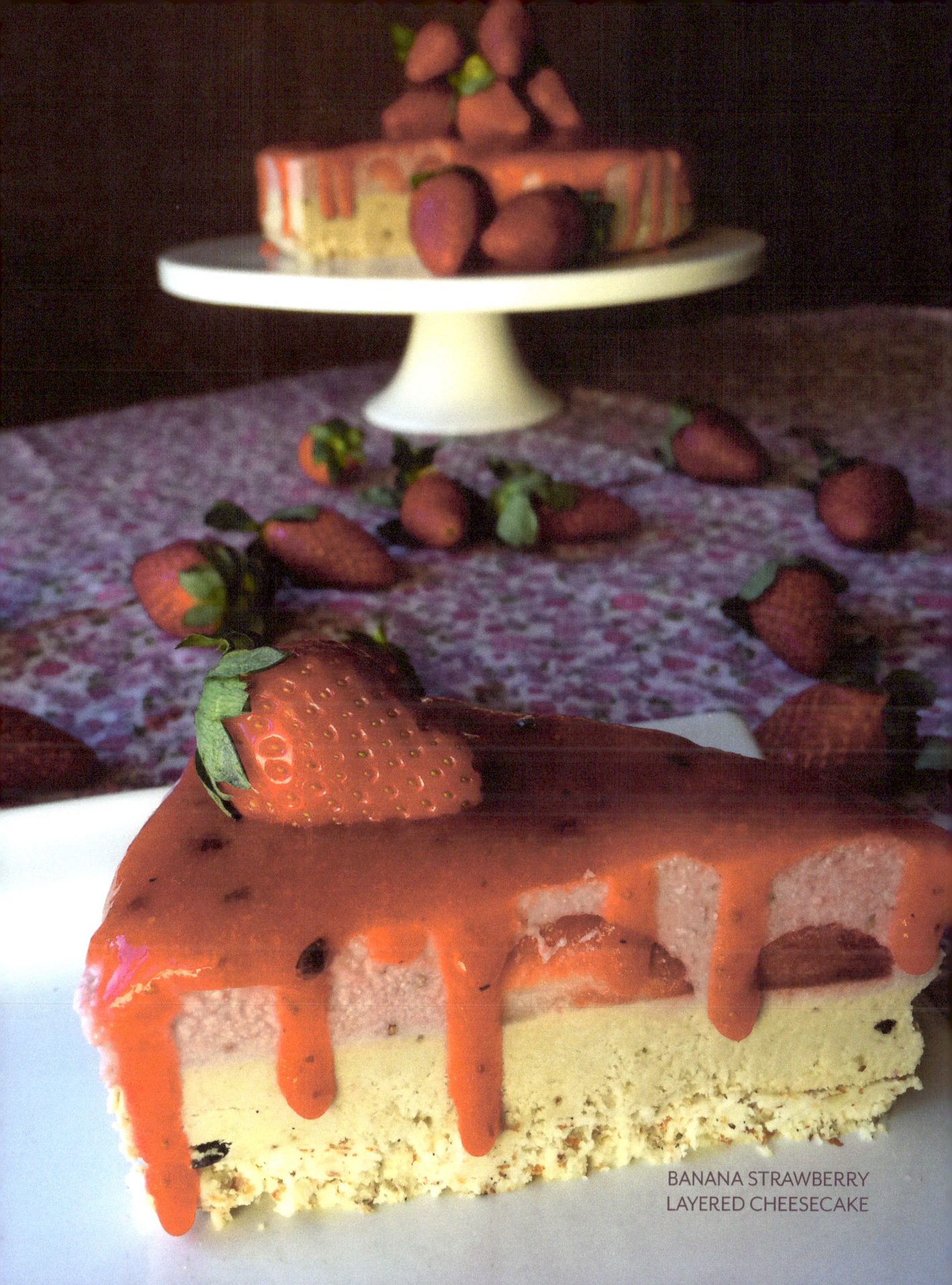
BANANA STRAWBERRY LAYERED CHEESECAKE

Chocolate Ganache Cakes with Orange Segments

INGREDIENTS

Base
- 1 cup macadamia nuts
- 3/4 cup almonds
- 50mls cacao butter (melted)
- 1/4 cup xylitol or 1 tbs stevia

Chocolate Ganache
- 1 cup of raw cashews (soaked for 3 hours)
- 3/4 cup cacao powder
- 3/4 cup rice malt syrup
- 3/4 cup coconut oil
- 1/4 cup coconut cream
- 1tbs vanilla extract
- a spin of the Himalayan salt grinder

Topping
- 2 Oranges or some other juicy fruit

METHOD

Base
Process all ingredients to bread crumb phase. Press mixture into 6 silicon cupcake molds or you can use hollow metal baking rings. Smooth out with the back of a spoon. Rest in freezer.

Chocolate Ganache
Blend all ingredients in food processor for 1 minute or until creamy. Pour into silicon molds on top of base. Allow to set in the freezer for an hour or two before garnishing with fruit.

Topping
Peel and cut oranges into segments, removing the white membrane. Remove cakes from silicon molds. Arrange fruit on top of each one. Enjoy.

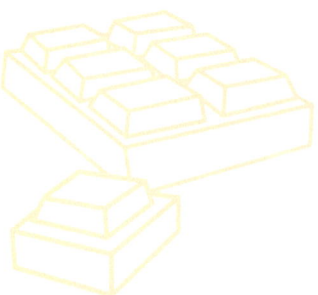

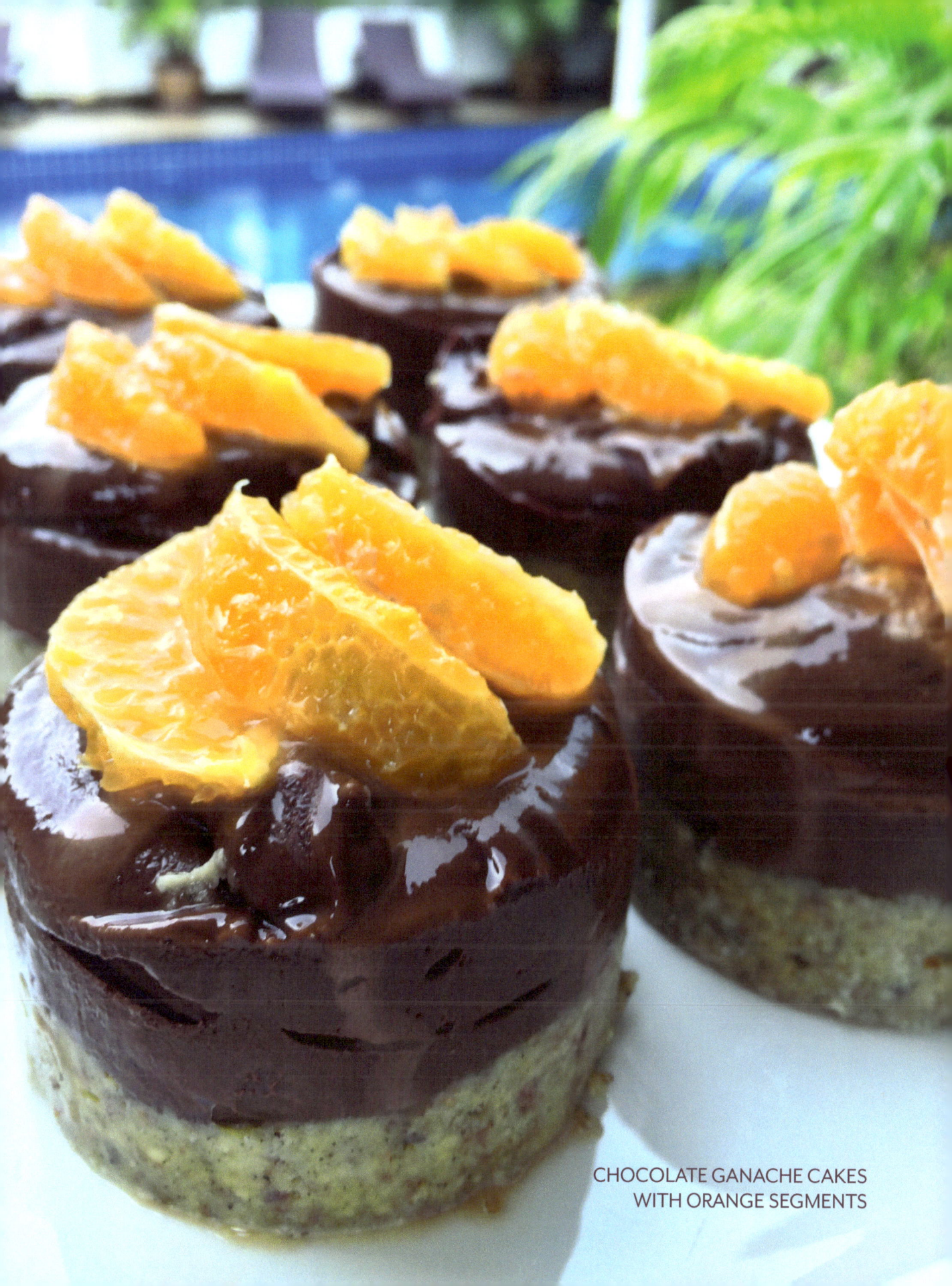

CHOCOLATE GANACHE CAKES
WITH ORANGE SEGMENTS

Lime Chocolate Cheesecake

This recipe is so good that it needs no introduction. If you can get your hands on some food grade lime essential oils like Doterra, then you will be jumping for joy when you taste this healthy treat.

INGREDIENTS

Base

- 1 cup almonds or almond meal pulp
- 1 cup macadamia nuts
- 1/4 cup coconut oil melted
- 1/4 cup cacao powder
- 1/2 - 1 tbs stevia
  (equivalent sweetness of 2 -3 tbs sugar – check the concentration of your brand)

Filling

- 2 cups cashews
  (soaked for 5 hours or overnight)
- 3/4 cups lime juice
- 1/2 cup coconut paste
- 1 1/2 cups rice malt syrup (or 1 cup rice malt syrup and stevia to taste)
- 1/4 cup coconut oil melted
- 5-10 drops Doeterra essential oil.
- lime rind for garnish.
  Note: Don't put lime rind in the cake, as it is bitter and will taste unpleasant.

METHOD

Base

Blend all dry ingredients in the food processor until the mixture forms a breadcrumb texture. Add oil and keep mixing until mixture can stick together when squeezed. Press into a lined and greased spring form tin. Ensure that the thickness is even and comes up at the sides. You may want to press it down with another piece of non-stick paper and use the back of a large spoon to get a smooth even consistency. Refrigerate.

Filling

Blend all ingredients except essential oils in a high-powered food processor until creamy. This may take a few minutes. Scrape down the sides of the bowl so that everything is incorporated. Taste, then add the essential oil a few drops at a time. Blend again and taste until you have the perfect flavor. Don't go overboard with the lime, as it can be bitter. Pour into the flan pan and chill for 5 hours in the freezer or overnight in the fridge. Garnish with lime zest or cacao nibs. Yum!

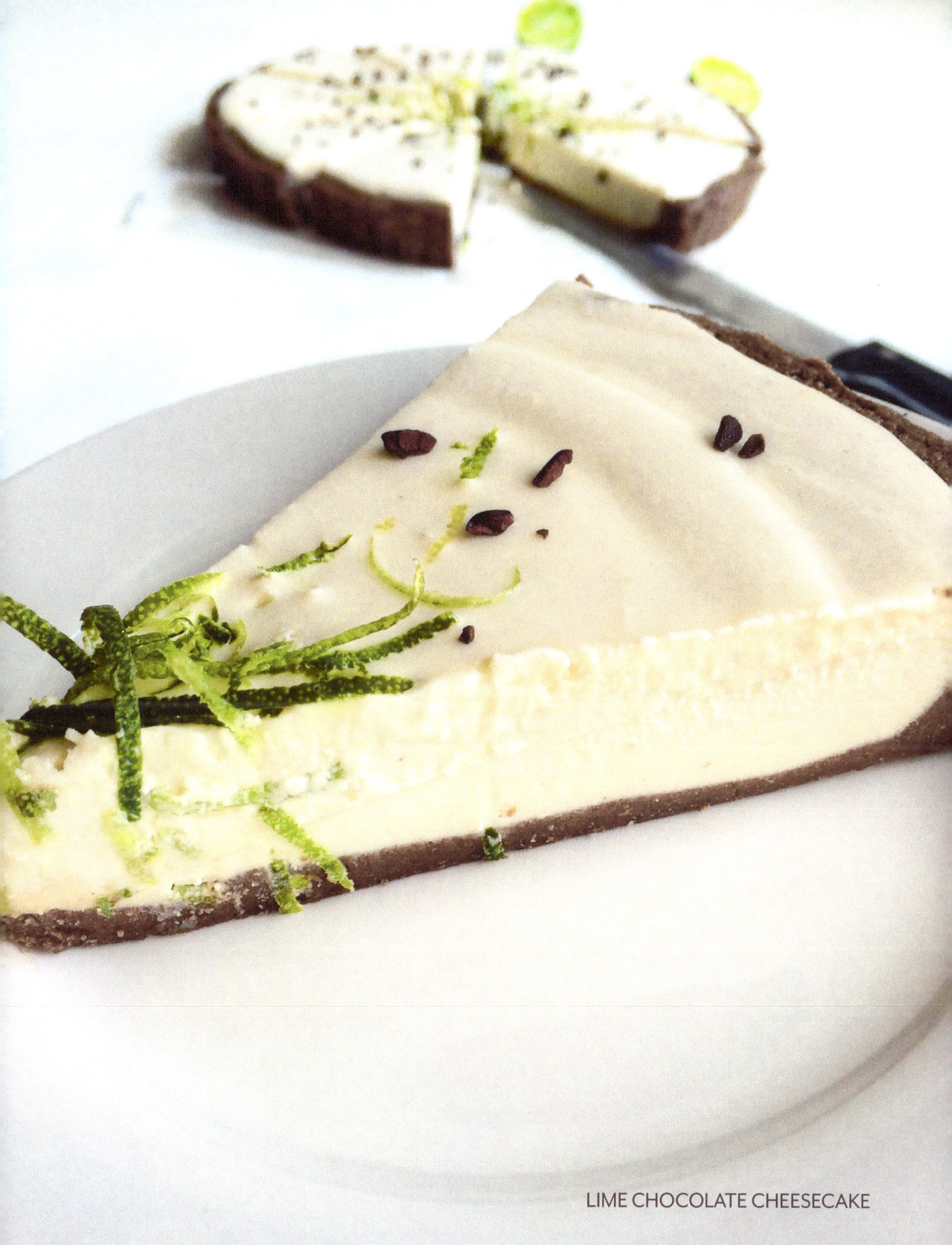

LIME CHOCOLATE CHEESECAKE

Mango Lychee Cheesecakes

INGREDIENTS

Base

- 1 1/2 cup almonds
- 1/2 cup dates
- 1/2 cup Angus Park apricots (or some tangy brand)
- 2 tbs coconut oil
- 1 tbs of lemon rind
- pinch of salt

Mango Lychee Layer

- 1 cup cashews (soaked)
- 2 mangoes, skinned and seeded
- 1/2 cup or 100g cacao butter (melted) or coconut paste
- 1/4 cup xylitol
- crackle of salt from the grinder
- lemongrass slices (optional)
- Garnish with 1/4 cup deseeded lychees (approx. 8) and mango slices.

METHOD

Base

Blend in a food processor. If you don't have a powerful food processor than you may need to blend the nuts first to a powder, then add the dried fruits one at a time. Squeeze mix into a ball, then press into a lined flan pan or spring form tin. Freeze.

Mango Lychee Layer

Blend all ingredients (except garnish) in a food processor until smooth. Adjust sweetness if desired by adding a little stevia. I use drops. Pour onto apricot base and freeze for 2 hours. Serve with slices of fresh mango and lychees.

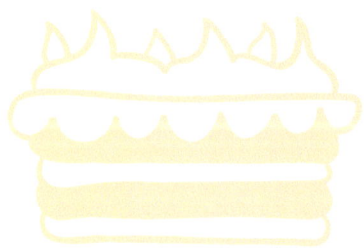

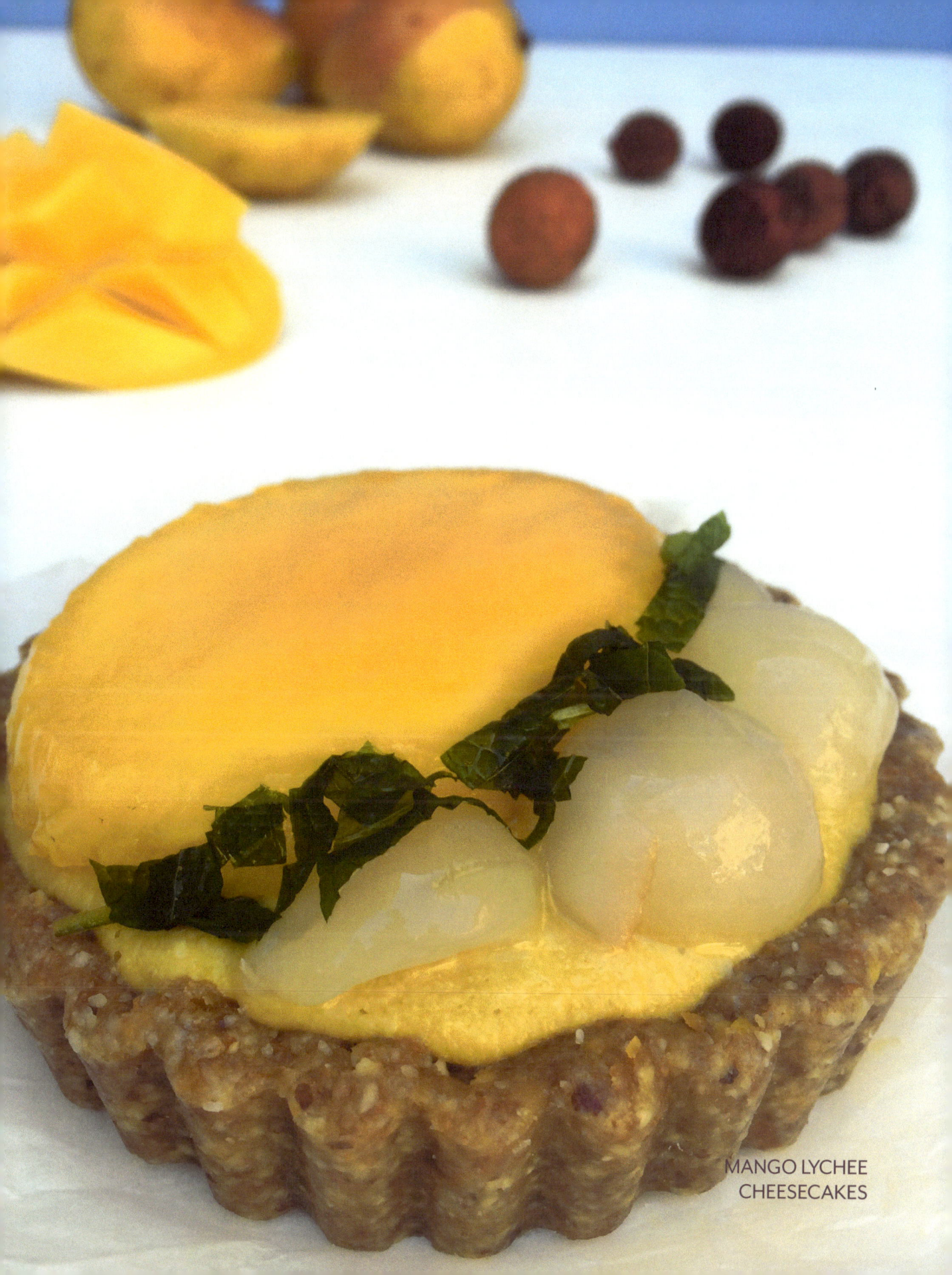

MANGO LYCHEE CHEESECAKES

White Chocolate Cherry Cheesecake

INGREDIENTS

Base

- 3/4 cups almonds
- 1 cup cashews
- 2 tbs cacao powder
- 1/4 cup coconut oil (melted)
- 1/2 cup rice malt syrup
- 1/2 cup desiccated coconut
- pinch of pink salt

Cheesecake Filling

- 2 cups of cashews (measure then soak these overnight)
- 1 1/2 cups of rice malt syrup
- 1/2 cup cacao butter melted (120g)
- 1/2 cup coconut oil melted
- 1 tbs vanilla essence
- 5 drops medicine flower white chocolate essence
- pinch of pink salt
- 2 cups of fresh cherries

METHOD

Base

Blend nuts and cacao in a high-powered food processor. Drizzle in syrup and oil. Crackle the salt grinder. Once dough texture has formed, roll it into a ball and press down on a lined spring form baking tin. Smooth with a wet hand. Place mixture in freezer to harden.

Cheesecake Filling

Blend cashew nuts and coconut oil until smooth and creamy. Add the vanilla essence and white chocolate essence to the melted cacao butter. Pour this into the food processor along with the rice malt syrup and continue processing. Add a pinch of salt to taste. Pour the mixture on top of the base and lightly press one cup of cherries into the white chocolate cheesecake until half submerged. Return to freezer to set for an hour. Remove and top with the remaining cherries and place in the fridge or freezer until ready to serve. Do not freeze the cherries.

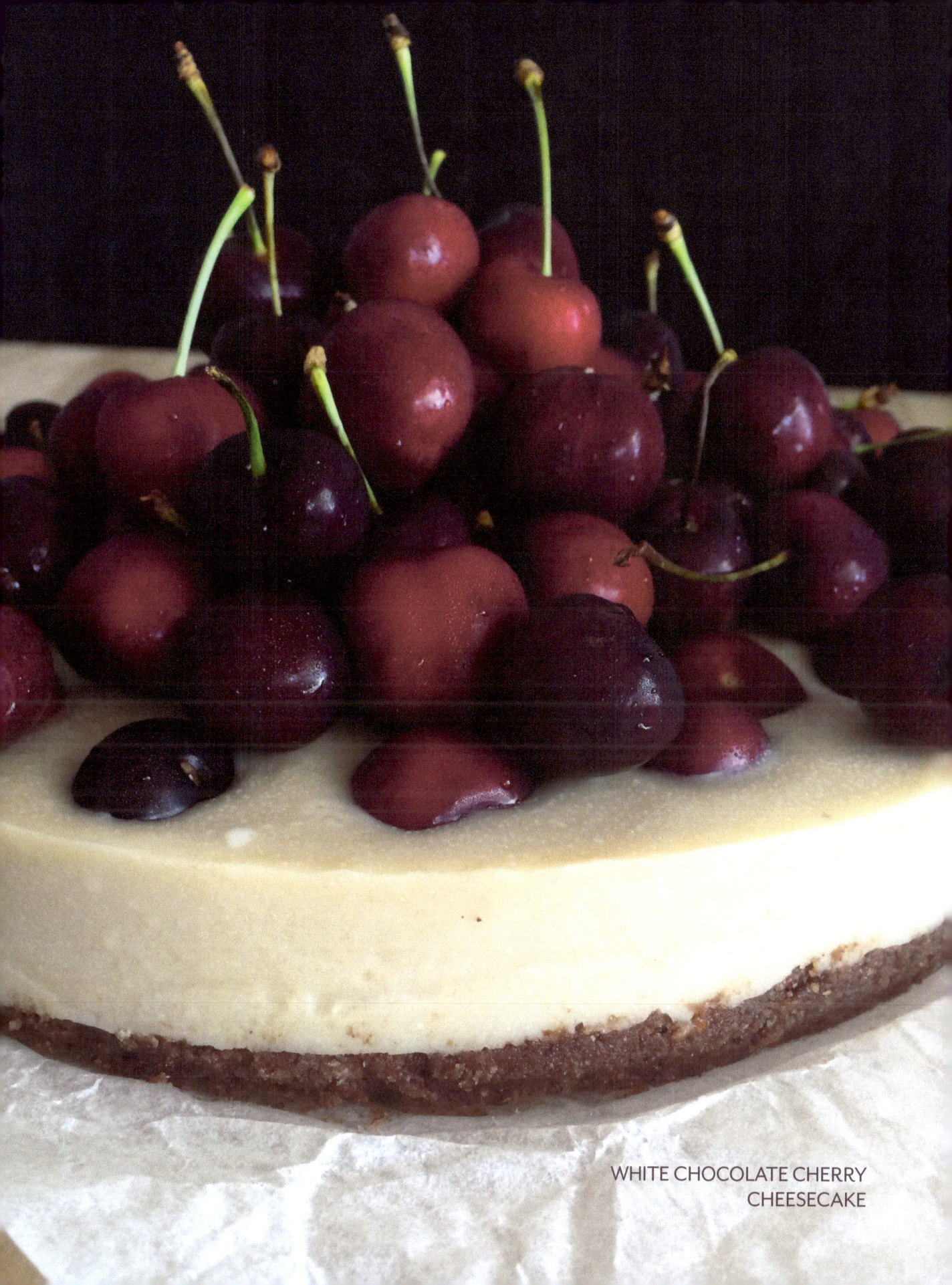

WHITE CHOCOLATE CHERRY
CHEESECAKE

White Chocolate Mango Cheesecake

This is such a striking looking dessert that makes perfect use of summer fruits. If mangoes and passionfruit aren't in season, then make something else. The key to this dessert's success is juicy ripe fruit. The white chocolate essence drops are optional, but I think they're the key to recreating an authentic chocolate taste, along with the cacao butter.

INGREDIENTS

Base

- » 1 cup almonds (or use leftover almond meal pulp)
- » 1/2 cup macadamia nuts
- » 1/4 cup coconut oil (melted)
- » 1/4 cup rice malt syrup
- » pinch of pink salt

Cheesecake Filling

- » 2 cups of cashews (measure then soak for 5 hours)
- » 1 cup rice malt syrup
- » 1/2 cup cacao butter melted (120g)
- » 1/2 cup coconut oil melted
- » 1/4 cup maple syrup
- » 6 white chocolate essence drops (Medicine Flower)
- » 1 – 2 tsp stevia to reach desired sweetness (or just add an extra 1/4 cup maple syrup)
- » pinch of pink salt
- » 2 – 3 ripe mangoes
- » 4 large passionfruit for garnish

METHOD

Base

Blend nuts in a high-powered food processor. Drizzle in syrup and oil. Crackle the salt grinder. Once dough has been formed, divide and roll it into 6 balls. Press down into each of the 6 metal cylinders or use 6 silicon cupcake molds. Smooth with a wet hand. Allow to set in freezer.

Cheesecake Filling

Blend together cashews, coconut oil and rice malt syrup. Adjust the sweetness with more maple or with stevia. Add a pinch of salt to taste. Pour half the mixture on top of the base until it half fills each mold and return to freezer to set for an hour.

Remove and place slices of the mango around the edges of the cylinders so that there are no air pockets. Once you have made a perimeter of mango, place the remaining mango slices in the middle of the white chocolate cheesecake. You don't want the mango to sink to the bottom, so make sure the cheesecake is firm before placing the mango slices on top. Pour over the remaining cheesecake mixture and place in the fridge to harden. Once firm, pop out each cake and top with passionfruit to serve.

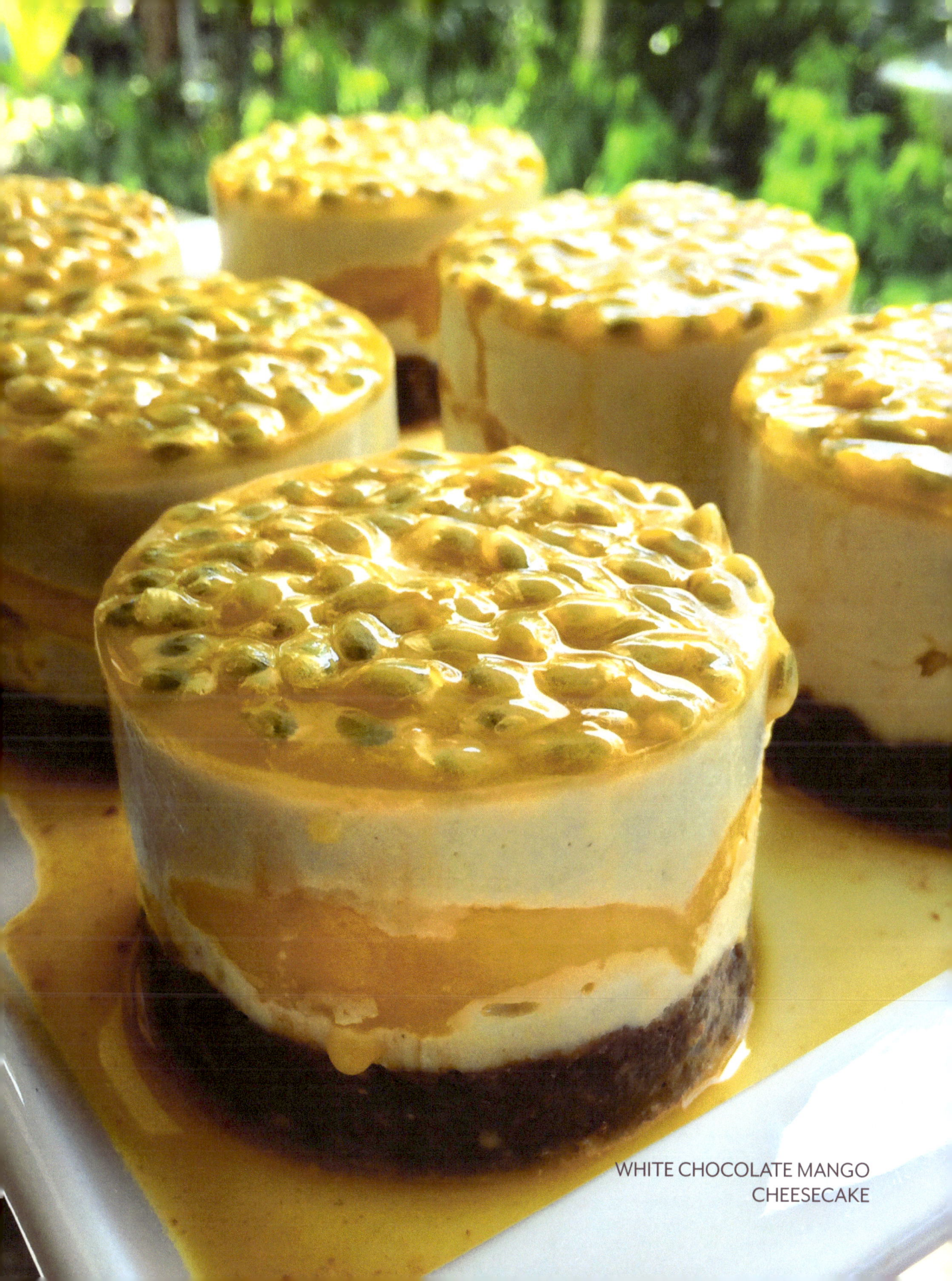
WHITE CHOCOLATE MANGO CHEESECAKE

Lemon, Lavender and Blueberry Cheesecakes

At first this may not seem like an obvious marriage. Isn't three a crowd? But I love the combination of lavender and blueberries because the fruit lends its fabulous color to match the hue of the lavender flavor, and lemon brings out the tartness of the fruit and gives a freshness to the healing lavender oil. I use culinary grade essential oils because it's easier than messing about with distilling the dried blooms, but you can use either. The base for this recipe is adapted from my lemon slice recipe. These photographs have not been boosted for color or undergone any editing. Just like my food, they are natural, raw and minimally processed. I hope you enjoy this raw dessert recipe that would sit just as comfortably on the vegan or paleo plate. Bon appetit!

INGREDIENTS

Base

- 3/4 cup almonds
- 1 cup dates pitted
- 3/4 cup desiccated coconut
- 3 tbs lemon rind (3 lemons)
- 1/2 cup lemon juice (or juice of 2 lemons)
- 2 tbs Lacuma powder (optional)
- 2 tbs coconut paste

Top Layer

- 1 cup cashews soaked for 5 hours or overnight
- 2 tbs lemon rind
- 1/2 cup coconut paste or oil
- 1/4 cup lemon juice
- 1 cup blueberries
- 3/4 cup rice malt syrup
- 3 drops of lavender essential oil (use a food grade oil like Doeterra)

METHOD

Base

Blend all dry ingredients in food processor first. Then blend in the wet ingredients until mixture forms a dough that sticks together. Divide into 8 and press into 8 silicon cupcake molds. Refrigerate.

Top Layer

In a food processor, blend nuts and coconut paste first until smooth. Add remaining ingredients, blending and scraping down the sides as you go. Once a creamy consistency is reached, pour nut and coconut mix onto lemon base. Freeze for several hours. Pop out of silicon molds when hard. Allow to defrost on bench 15 minutes before serving.

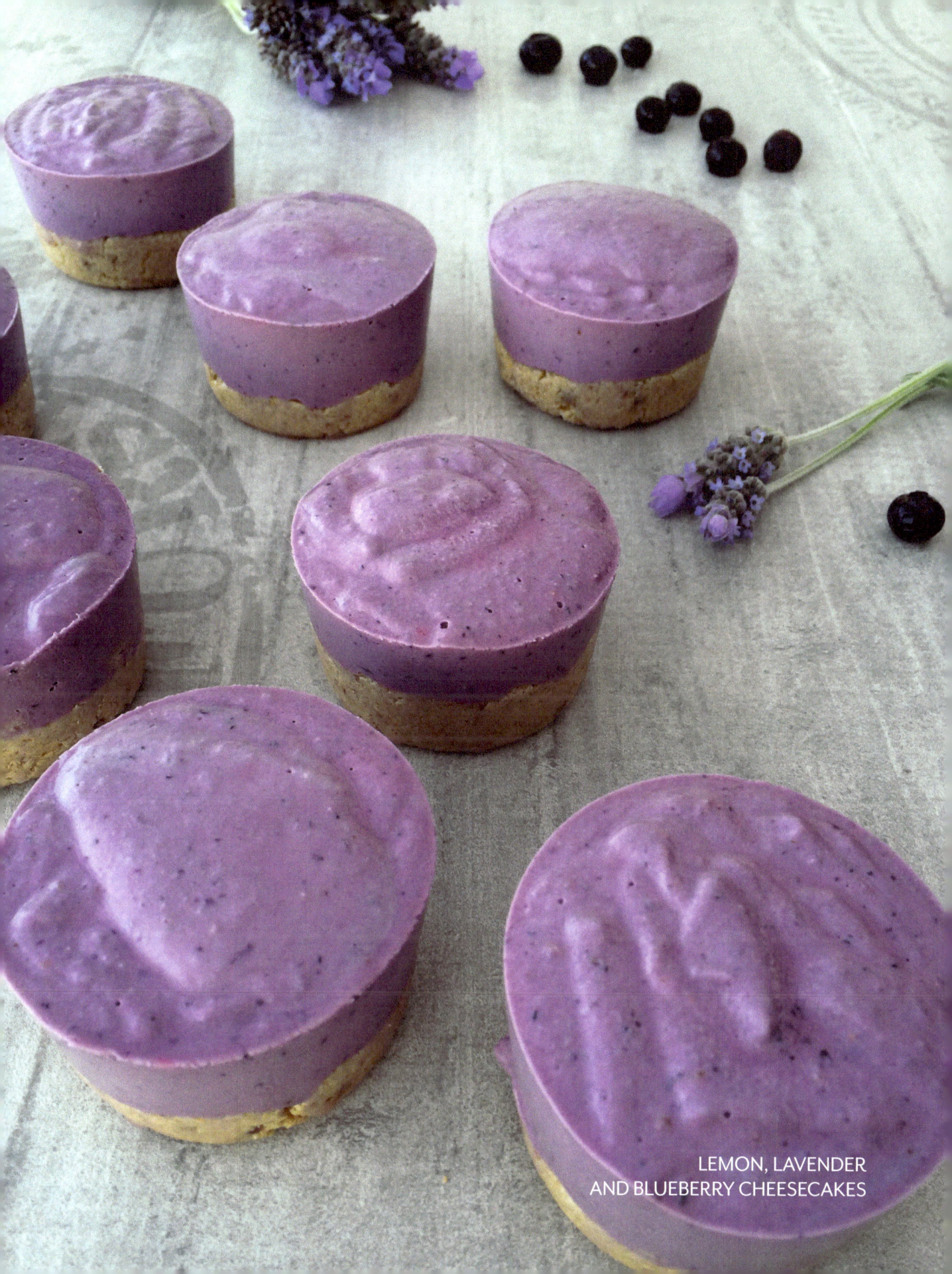

LEMON, LAVENDER AND BLUEBERRY CHEESECAKES

Raspberry and Pomegranate Mini Cheesecakes

The flavors of coconut and lemon set the stage for the delicate and juicy morsels of raspberries. This is a great recipe if you are over dates. There are no dates here.

I like the idea of having small cakes on hand to take to friends' homes for dinner or as a treat for only a few people. You can keep the slices naturally small. It's all about portion control. These aren't individual serves, mind you. I've been known to slice one of these up to serve 6 people. If you don't have baby flan pans like the ones pictured here, you can use cupcake molds or a regular cake tin.

INGREDIENTS

Base

- » 1 cup desiccated coconut
- » 1/2 cup macadamia nuts
- » zest and juice of 1 lemon
- » 1 tbs rice malt syrup

Filling

- » 1 1/2 cups cashews (presoak overnight in water)
- » 3/4 cup coconut cream
- » 2/3 cup rice malt syrup
- » 1/2 cup coconut paste (or oil)
- » 1 tbs lemon zest
- » 3/4 cup frozen raspberries (stir these in at the end)

For Garnish

- » 1/2 cup fresh raspberries
- » 1/4 cup pomegranate seeds (optional)

METHOD

Base

Blend all ingredients in food processor until mixture sticks together in a ball. Press into a small flan pan lined with baking paper. Use the back of a spoon to create a smooth even layer.

Filling

Blend cashews, coconut cream, rice malt syrup, coconut paste and lemon zest until smooth and creamy. Scrape down sides as you go and keep blending. Open pomegranate and release seeds. Pour any juice into the cheesecake blend. Gently stir in raspberries by hand. If they are frozen, they may start to streak their lovely red juice across the white cheesecake mix. Fabulous! Pour onto prepared bases. Chill in freezer for an hour or until set. Top with pomegranate seeds and fresh raspberries.

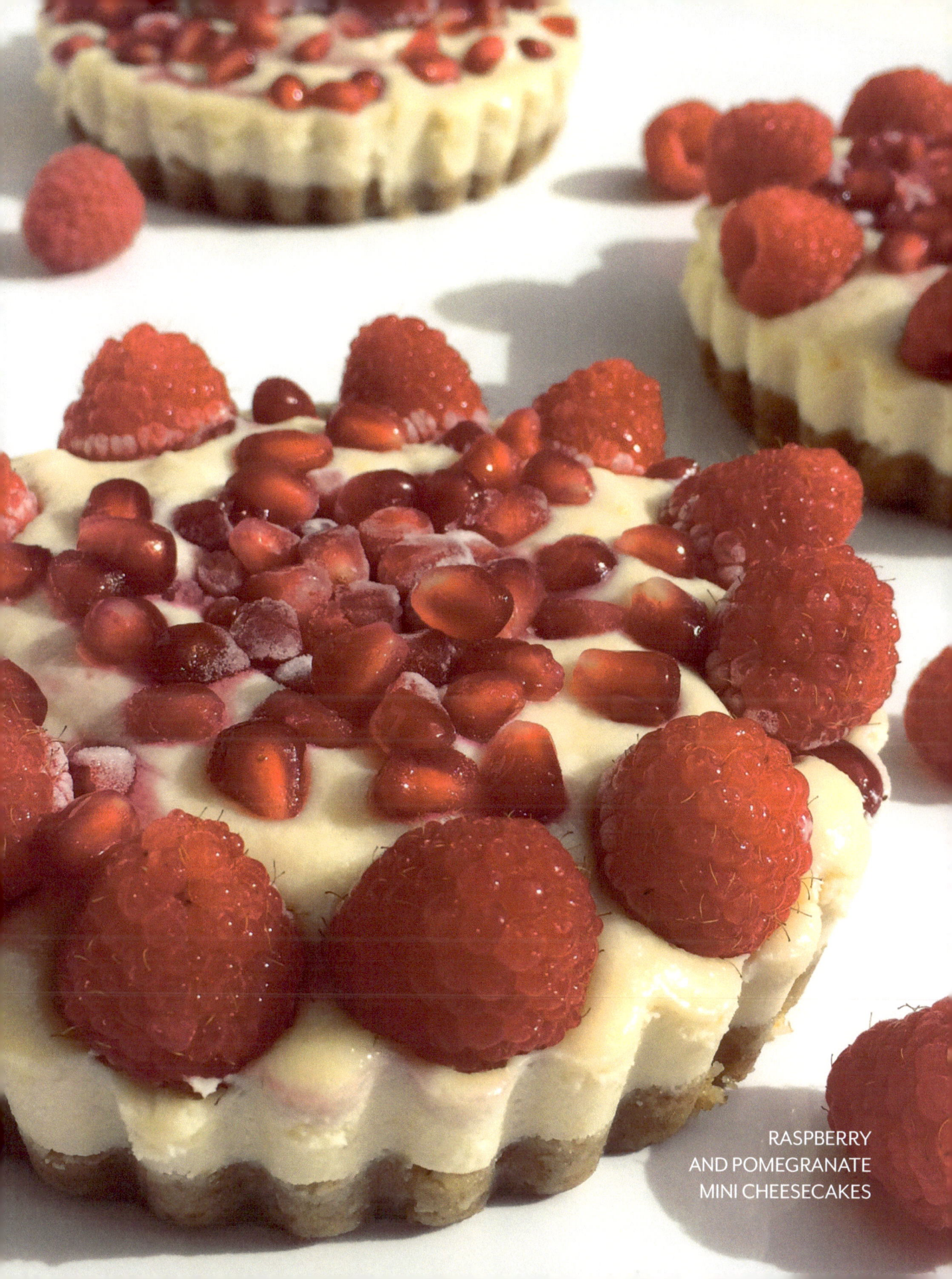

RASPBERRY AND POMEGRANATE MINI CHEESECAKES

Salted Caramel Cream Cake

I wanted to make something small but delicious. Many of the raw dessert recipes can become quite expensive when you make large celebration cakes, and not everyone has a family of 10 to feed. I've used two baby-sized tins with a diameter of 11cm (4 1/2 inches). If you make the quantity too small, there may not be enough volume for the blades to pick up and blend. This is best made with the small bowl in your food processor or similar high powered but small blender such as a Kenwood hand mixer with a bowl attachment.

INGREDIENTS

Base

- 3/4 cup macadamia nuts
- 1/3 cup desiccated coconut
- 1/4 cup packed dates
- 1 tbs cacao powder
- 1 tbs water

Caramel

- 1/2 cup pure peanut butter or almond butter
- 1/2 cup or 8 Medjool dates
- 1/4 cup rice malt syrup
- 1/4 cup coconut oil
- 1 cup coconut cream (2 x 1/2 cup)
- 1 tbs vanilla extract
- 1 tsp Maldon sea salt
- 1 - 2 bananas to serve

METHOD

Base

Blend nuts, cacao and coconut until crumbly, in a small bowl food processor. Add in dates and water and continue mixing until it forms a ball. Divide into two balls. Press into 2 small cake tins lined with baking paper. Chill.

Caramel

Blend nut butter, dates, 1/4 cup rice malt syrup, coconut oil, 1/2 cup coconut cream, salt and vanilla until smooth in the small bowl of the food processor. When smooth with no lumps of dates remaining, scoop out 1/2 a cup of this mixture and reserve for the topping later.

Then to the main caramel mixture, add an additional 1/2 cup coconut cream to the caramel mix. Blend again in food processor until creamy consistency. Pour into cake tin. Refrigerate or freeze until set (1 - 2 hours). Top with slices of fresh banana. Arrange them in a circle starting with the circumference first and then overlapping and working your way toward the center. Top with the left over caramel.

A NOTE ABOUT DATES: When I need to recreate a caramel flavor, I almost always use Medjool dates. They are soft and chewy and much easier to blend, leaving a smooth caramel texture. When I want to use dates to sweeten a cake base or make energy balls, I'll use the regular kind of dried dates because they are much cheaper. I would recommend using Medjool dates wherever possible as they have a superior taste and texture, but if you can't get your hands on them, you could soak the regular dried dates in a little warm water to soften them. Then use them to make your caramel.

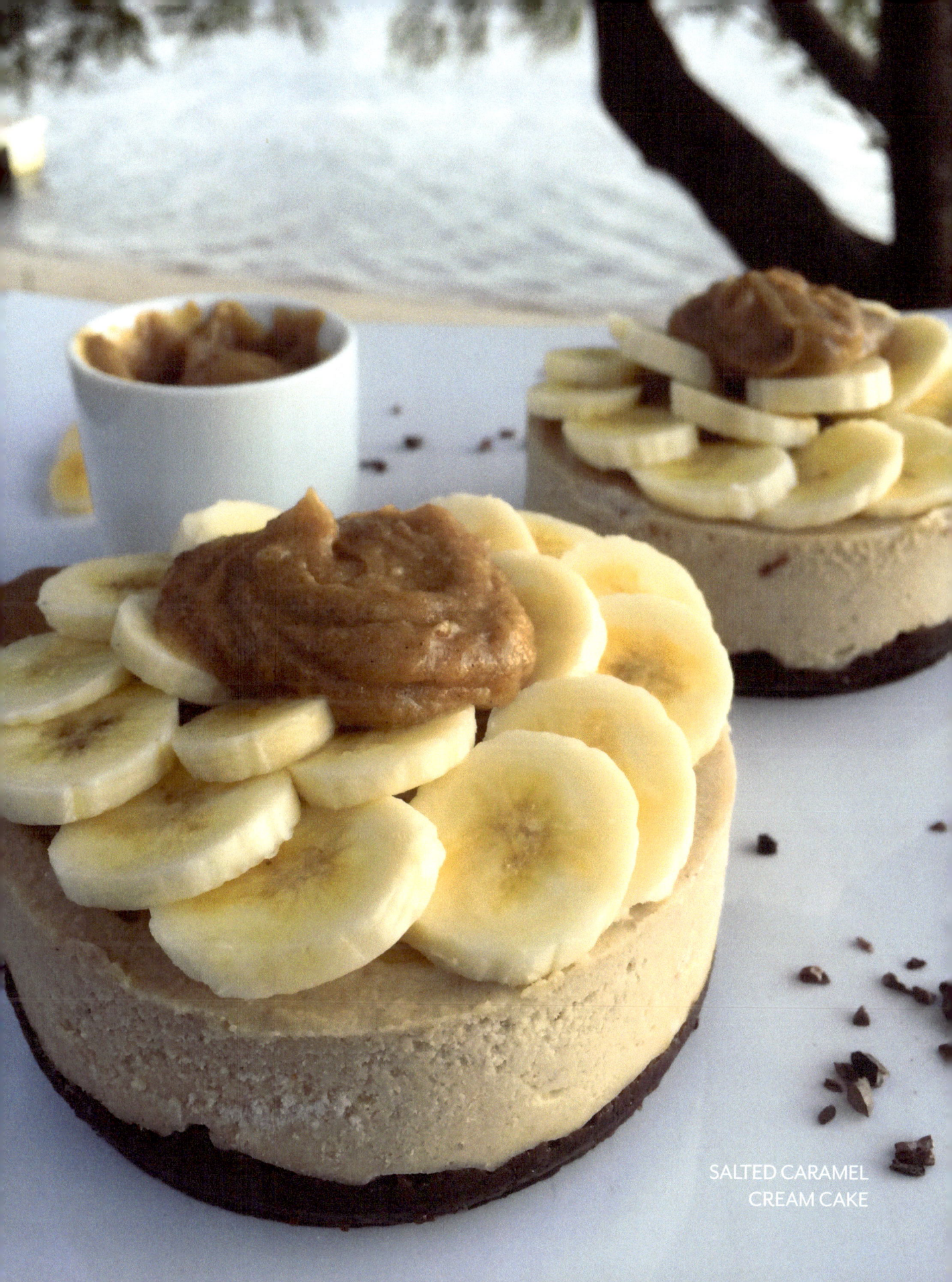

SALTED CARAMEL CREAM CAKE

Cherry Lemon Cheesecake

INGREDIENTS

Base
- 2 cups cashews or almonds
- 1 cup desiccated coconut
- 1 cup dates
- 1/4 cup coconut oil

Filling
- 2 cups cashews (soaked)
- 1/2 cup coconut oil
- 1/2 cup coconut butter
- 3/4 cup lemon juice
- 1 tbs lemon rind
- 3/4 cup rice malt syrup
- 1/2 cup deseeded cherries (fresh or frozen)

METHOD

Base
Blend nuts and coconut in food processor. Add dates and coconut oil while motor is still running. Once mixture starts to clump together or can form a ball when pressed together, press into a round spring-form tin lined with baking paper. Refrigerate.

Filling
Blend and pour on base.

Cherry Swirl
Purée 1/2 cup cherries and pour on top of cheesecake. Take a knife and swirl the mixture with the lighter colored one. Press in another cup of fresh cherries.

Place in freezer to set until firm but not frozen. (Maybe 2 hours.)

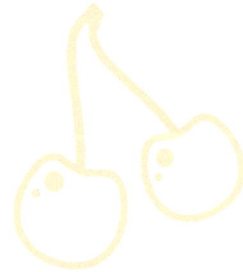

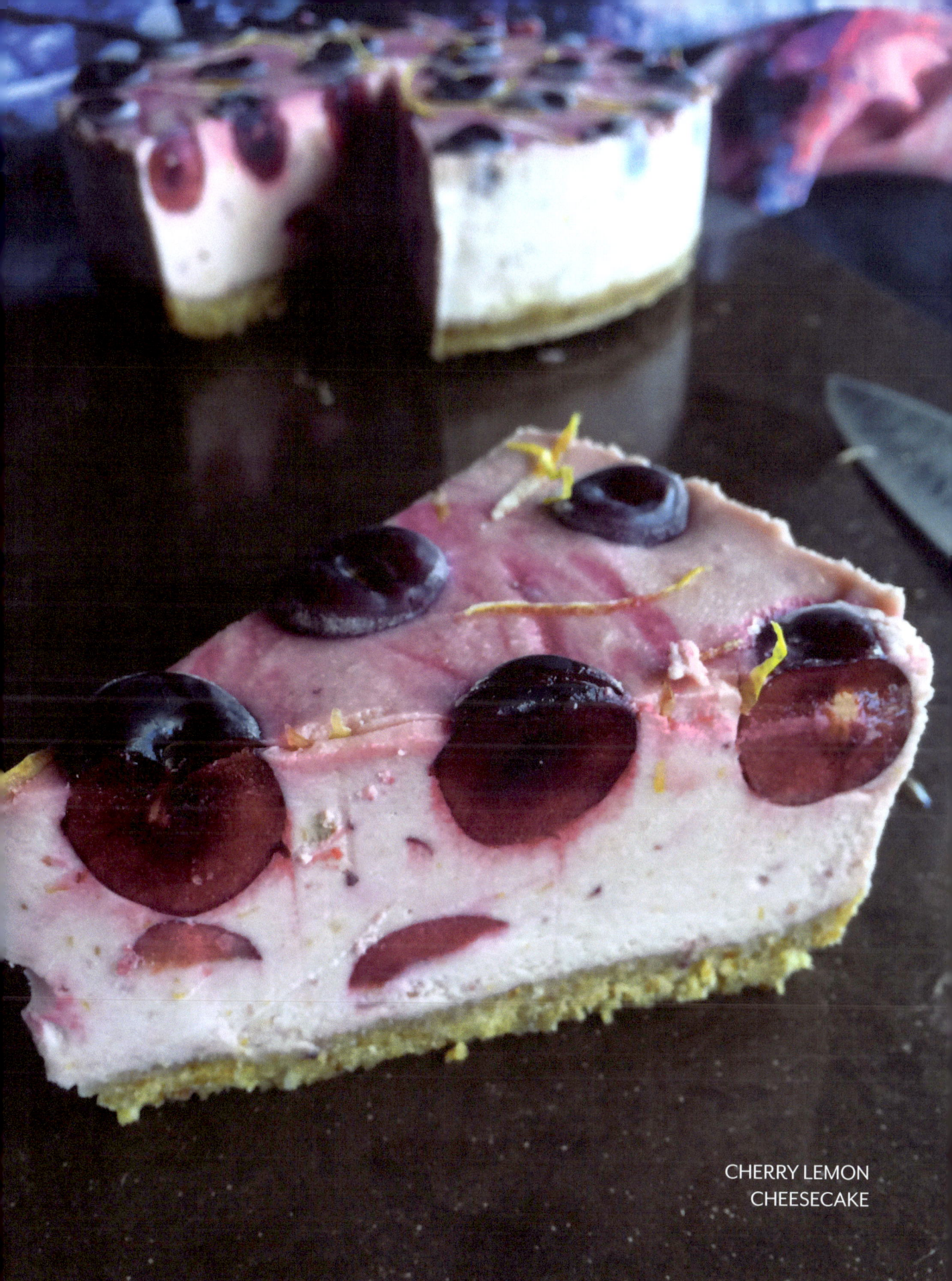

CHERRY LEMON CHEESECAKE

Chaimisu

This is a Chai layered mousse cake, inspired by Tiramisu. The recipe may seem lengthy but it's not really very complicated. However, it does require time for the layers to set.

INGREDIENTS

Chai Almond Milk

- 1 cup almonds (measure them dry then presoak)
- 3 cups water
- 1/4 tsp clove powder
- 3 cardamom pods
- 1 tsp cinnamon
- 1/4 tsp nutmeg
- 6 stevia drops
  (you can also use green stevia powder which is its most natural form)

Vanilla Almond Milk

- 1 cup almonds (measure then presoak)
- 3 cups of water
- 1 tbs pure vanilla extract or 2 whole vanilla beans, scraped
- 6 vanilla stevia drops

Base

- 3 cups spiced almond meal (use the leftover pulp from making the milk – it's the right amount)
- 2 cups dates
- 1/3 cup coconut oil
- 1/4 cup coconut flour
- salt

METHOD

Begin by making the chai and vanilla almond milks. It's important to make your own so you can use the almond pulp for the base. Use Agar Agar, vege-set or some other vegan gelling agent that works like gelatine. Agar works best by putting it into cold water and bringing it to the boil.

Chai Almond Milk

Blend all ingredients for several minutes until all almonds are pulverised. Strain off liquid through a nut bag suspended over a tall jug. Squeeze pulp to extract all the liquid. Reserve almond pulp for base. Then make vanilla almond milk.

Vanilla Almond Milk

Blend all ingredients in a blender for a minute or two. Strain liquid through a nut bag. Reserve almond pulp for base.

Base

Process all ingredients in food processor until crumbly and combined. Press into a lined square tin with a removable base. I used a large 10inch square pan (25.5cm x 25.5cm) Refrigerate.

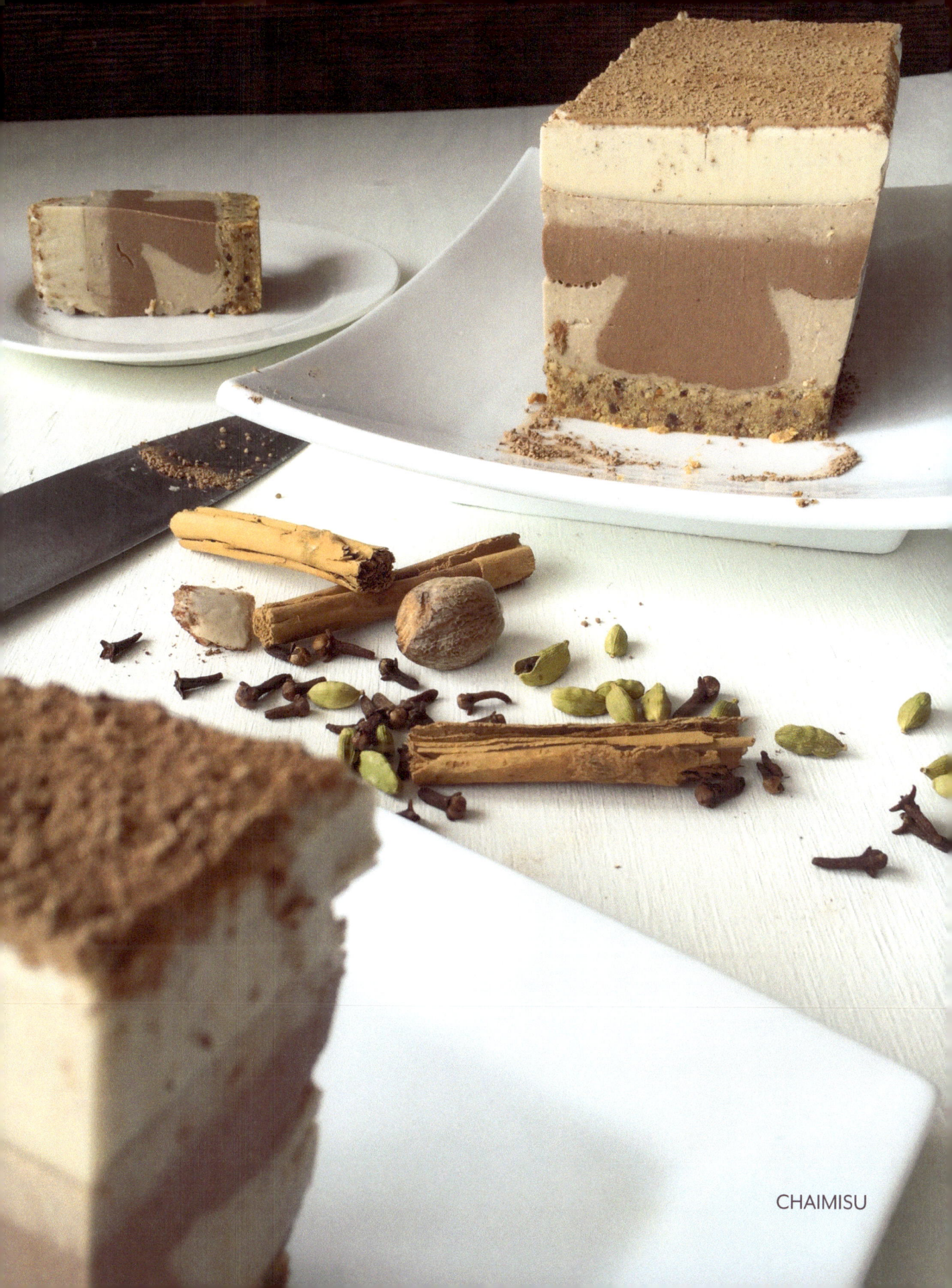

CHAIMISU

Chai Mousse Layer

- 2 cups chai almond milk
- 2 cups coconut cream
- 8 dates
- 1 cardamon pod
- 1 tbs vanilla
- 1/2 tsp cinnamon
- 1/4 tsp nutmeg
- 2 tbs agar agar (or vegan gelatine substitute) dissolved in 1/2 cup cold water, then brought to the boil.

Chocolate Layer

- 1 cup chai almond milk
- 1 cup vanilla almond milk
- 1 cup coconut cream
- 1/2 cup cacao powder
- 1/2 cup coconut oil or melted cacao butter
- 1/2 cup rice malt syrup
- extra stevia drops to sweeten
- 1 tbs agar agar stirred into 1/4 cup boiling water

Top Vanilla Layer

- 2 cups vanilla almond milk
- 2 cups coconut cream
- 1 tbs vanilla essence/ extract
- 1/2 cup rice malt syrup
- 2 tbs agar agar which has been dissolved in 1/2 cup boiling water (follow manufacturer's instructions)

Chai Mousse Layer

Blend all ingredients except agar agar in blender until smooth. With the motor running, pour in the dissolved agar agar. Keep blending for another minute. Pour the mixture into the tin on top of the base layer and chill until set.

Go on to make the chocolate layer.

Chocolate Layer

Blend all ingredients, except agar, in a blender and adjust for sweetness. While the motor is still running, pour in the agar mix and keep blending. Allow to cool before pouring on top of the chai mousse layer. Note: It's important to wait until the mixture is set so the layers don't blend. Return tray to fridge until chocolate layer is set.

Top Vanilla Layer

Blend all ingredients except agar agar in blender until smooth. With the motor running, pour in the dissolved agar. Keep blending for another minute. Pour the mixture into the tin on top of the chocolate mousse layer and chill until set, which will take several hours or overnight. Dust with cacao powder.

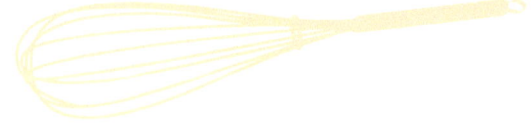

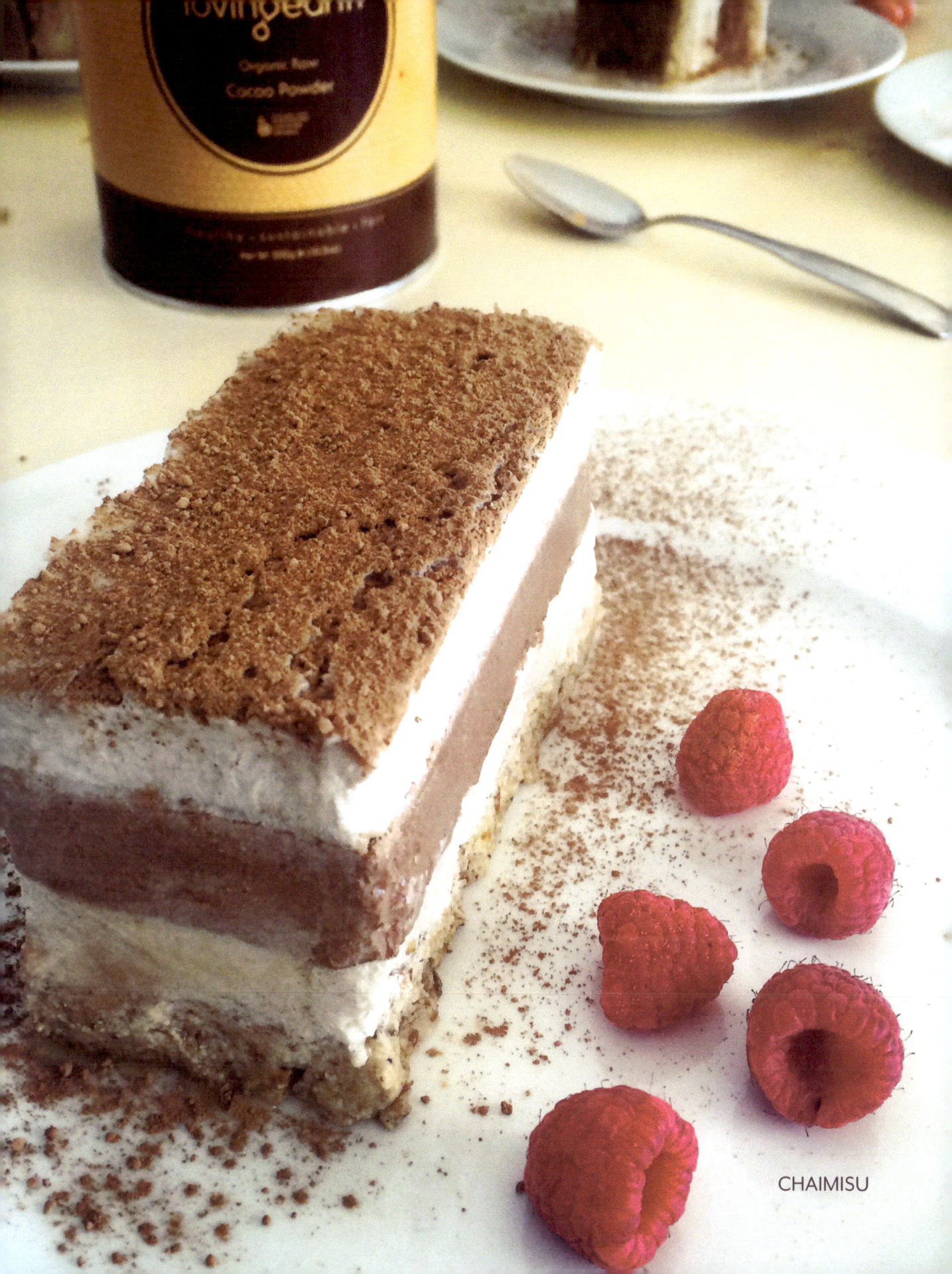
CHAIMISU

Spiced Apple Cakes with Cream

These are the perfect little cakes to have for afternoon tea. Adjust the spice level if you are not a big fan of cloves. The big tip is to use a sweet walnut. Some of the cheaper brands can taste bitter. I use Californian walnuts. If you are not sure, go on a little taste-testing spree and try some different brands and you will soon see the difference.

INGREDIENTS

Base

- 2 cups walnuts
- 2 tbs cinnamon powder
- 1 tsp clove powder
- 1/4 cup rice malt syrup
- 1/2 cup sultanas
- 2 tbs coconut oil melted
- 1 tsp stevia powder

Filling

- 4 green apples
- 1 tbs lemon juice
- 1 heaped cup of walnuts
- 1 – 2 tbs cinnamon powder
- 1 tsp clove powder
- 2 cardamom pods
- 1 -2 tsp stevia
- 1/4 cup rice malt syrup
- 200mls coconut cream or yoghurt (to serve)

METHOD

Base

Blend nuts spices and stevia in the food processor until crumbly. Add sultanas, oil and rice malt syrup and continue blending until the mixture forms a ball of dough. Taste, add more stevia if needed, and blend. Press mix evenly into the base of 6 silicon cupcake molds. Use a spoon to ensure that it is of even thickness. Allow to set in the freezer while you make the filling.

Filling

Grate apples into a large bowl and squeeze over lemon juice. Blend nuts and spices in a food processor until the mixture resembles bread crumbs. Drizzle in rice malt syrup and add stevia while the food processor is still running. Add grated apple and pulse until just mixed. Press mix into the cake molds. Serve with a vanilla coconut yoghurt or cream.

If you'd like this recipe sweeter, then adjust the stevia, not the rice malt syrup as it will affect the texture. I've used the green unprocessed stevia in this recipe. Since stevia varies greatly in sweetness, depending on which brand you buy, add a little at a time, or omit if you don't need it.

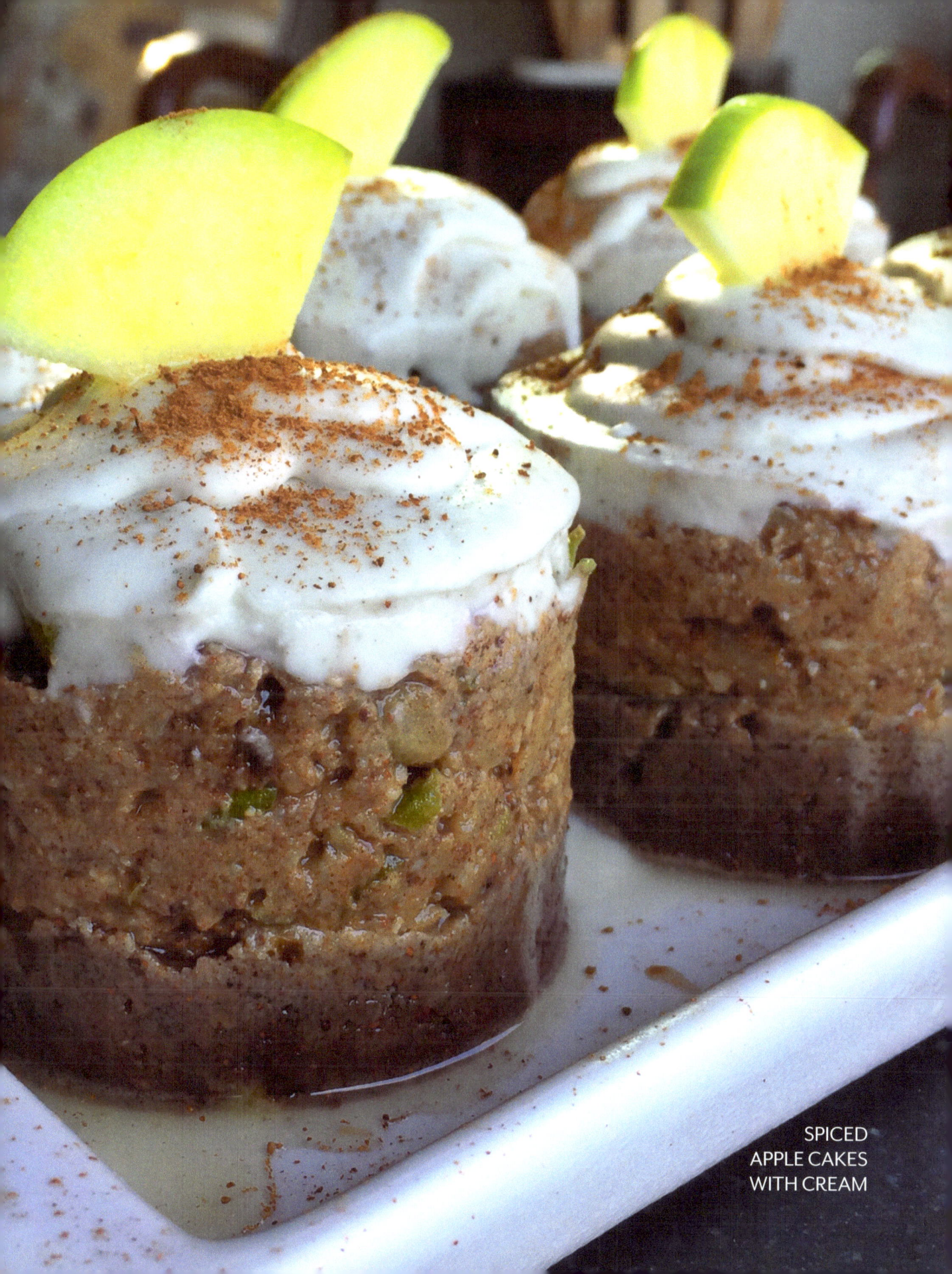

SPICED APPLE CAKES WITH CREAM

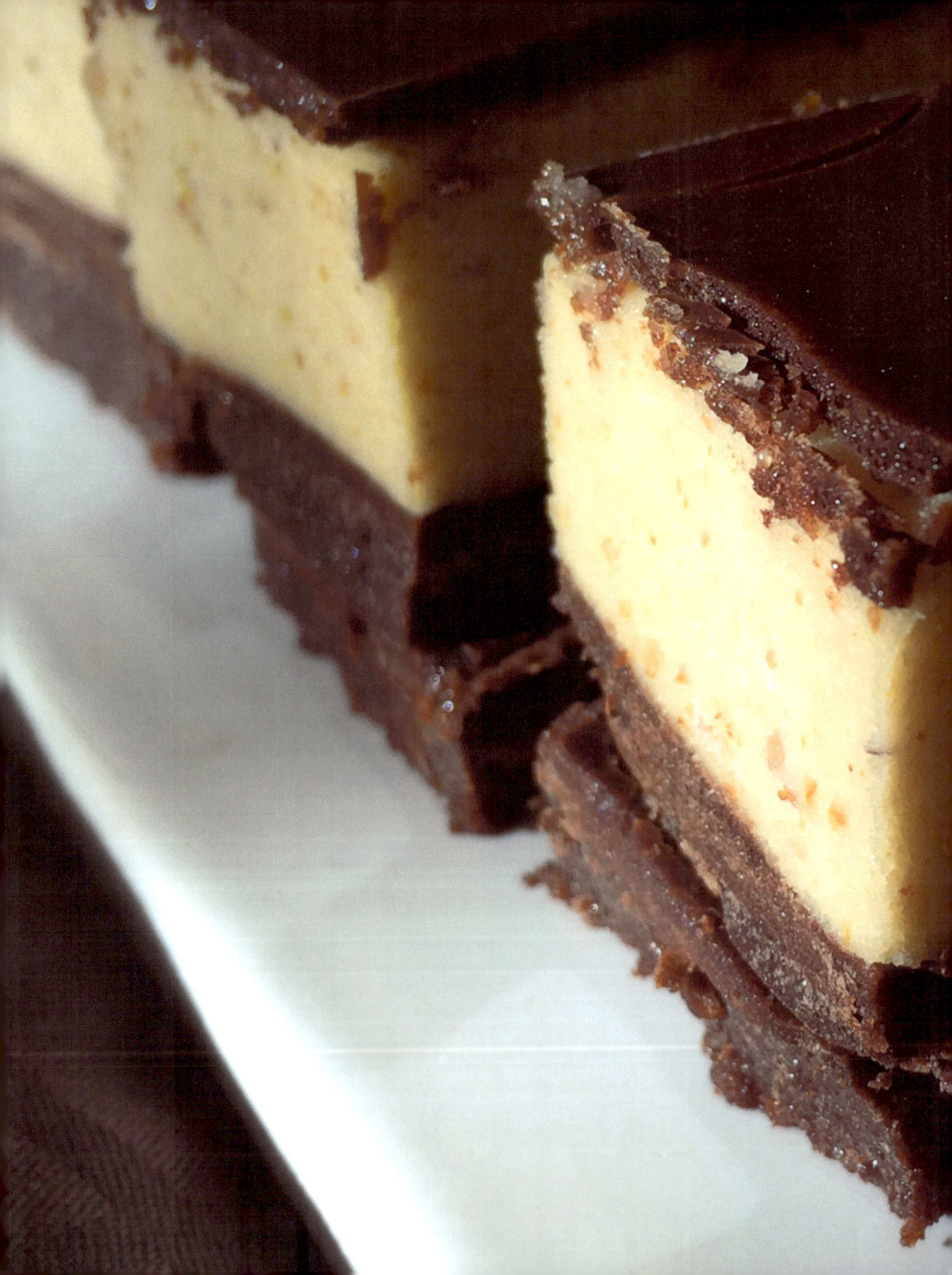

Chocolate & Fudge

Mint Chocolate Thins

This minty chocolate is packed full of antioxidants, and an energizing blend of Ormus green superfood powders, berries and fresh mint. Ormus is reported to be healing and gives the body and mind an uplifting boost of energy. Some others report on its magical mind opening abilities. You can quite easily halve this recipe to make a smaller batch but it's so delicious that I make up a large quantity and just store it in the freezer to satisfy my need for a chocolatey energy hit. I love the chewy texture of this mint thin.

INGREDIENTS

- 1 cup raw cacao powder
- 1 cup raw cacao butter melted
- 3/4 cup rice malt syrup or maple syrup
- 2 tbs green powder (try spirulina, barley grass, Ormus greens or another blend)
- 5 - 10 drops of pure peppermint essential oils

METHOD

Shave the cacao butter with a sharp knife into shards or smaller pieces. Place in a bowl that is inside a larger bowl of hot water. This will melt the cacao butter. Once liquid, mix in the cacao powder, green powder, and syrup. Add 5 peppermint essence drops and mix well by hand before tasting. Add more until desired flavor is reached. I use about 10 drops. Line a baking tray with baking paper and pour the chocolate onto the tray and spread out evenly. Garnish with a handful of fresh mint leaves (the more the better). Refrigerate or freeze until set. Then slice into thin squares. I love using a tray as opposed to molds, as it's quicker and results in a peppermint thin that reminds me of the classic 'after dinner mint' or After Eights.

Garnish with 1-2 tbs goji berries and 1-2 tbs raw pistachio nuts and a sprinkle of salt to make a festive Christmas looking chocolate.

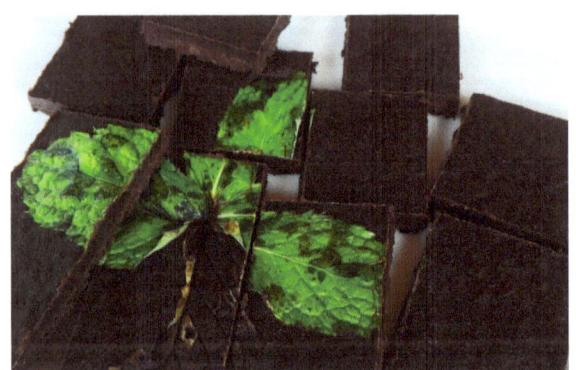

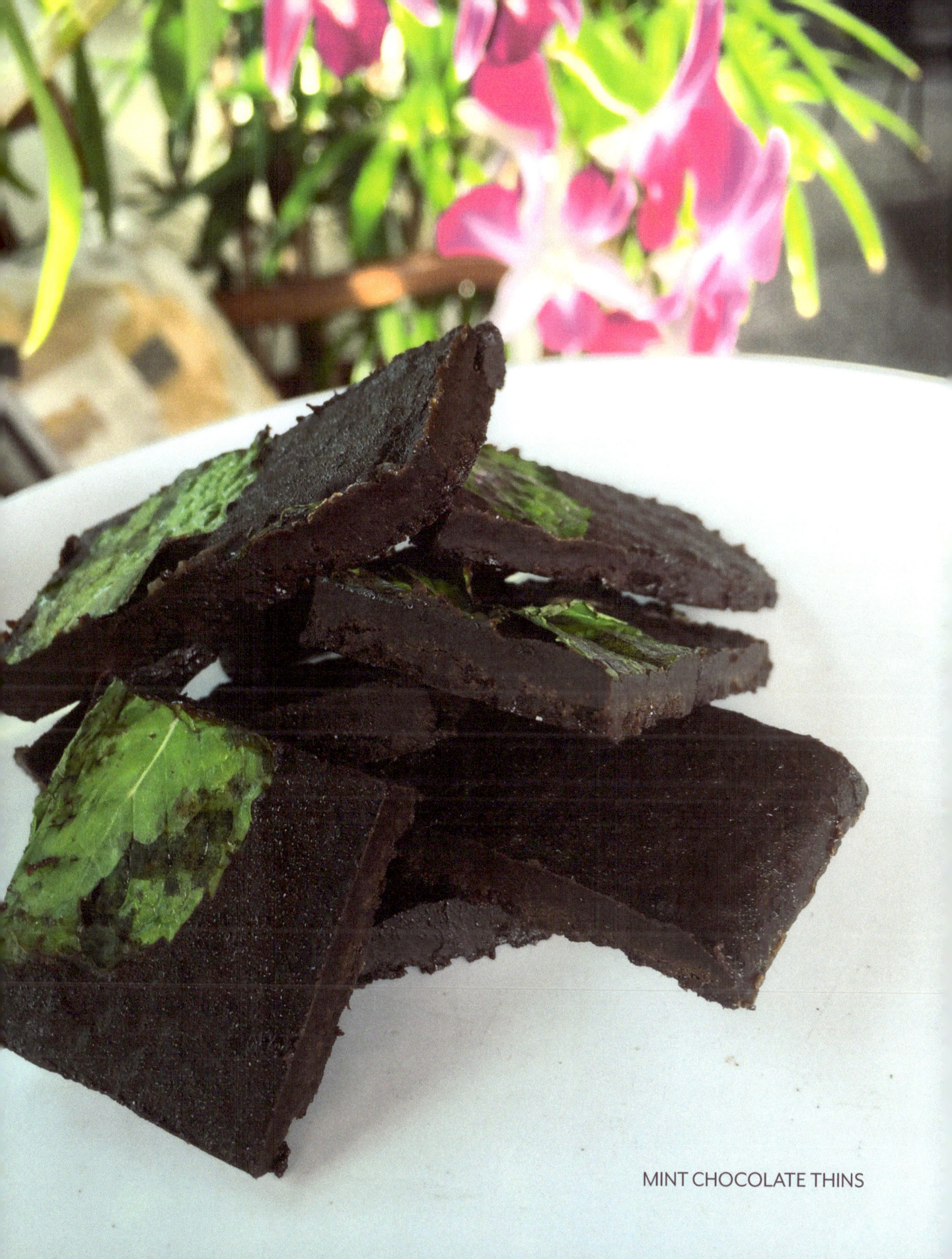

MINT CHOCOLATE THINS

White Chocolate Chunk

Make these small chocolate bites by using the ice-cube trays from your freezer. Use the traditional cube or some fancy ones with shapes. Press a whole fresh cherry into the middle and you have a cute little sweet, perfect for petit fours at the end of a meal.

INGREDIENTS

- 1/2 cup cacao butter (melted) about 120g
- 1/4 cup cashews (soaked in water for a few hours or overnight)
- 3 tbs pure maple syrup
- 1 tsp vanilla extract
- fresh cherries (about 12)

METHOD

An easy way to melt the cacao butter is to shave off shards of cacao butter from the whole block with a sharp knife, then melt it inside a jar sitting in a bowl of hot water. Blend cashews and cacao butter in the small bowl of your food processor until smooth. Pour in maple syrup and vanilla and mix until well combined. Pour evenly into ice cube trays and press in a cherry until 3/4 submerged. Refrigerate until set.

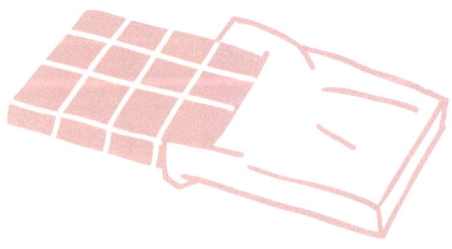

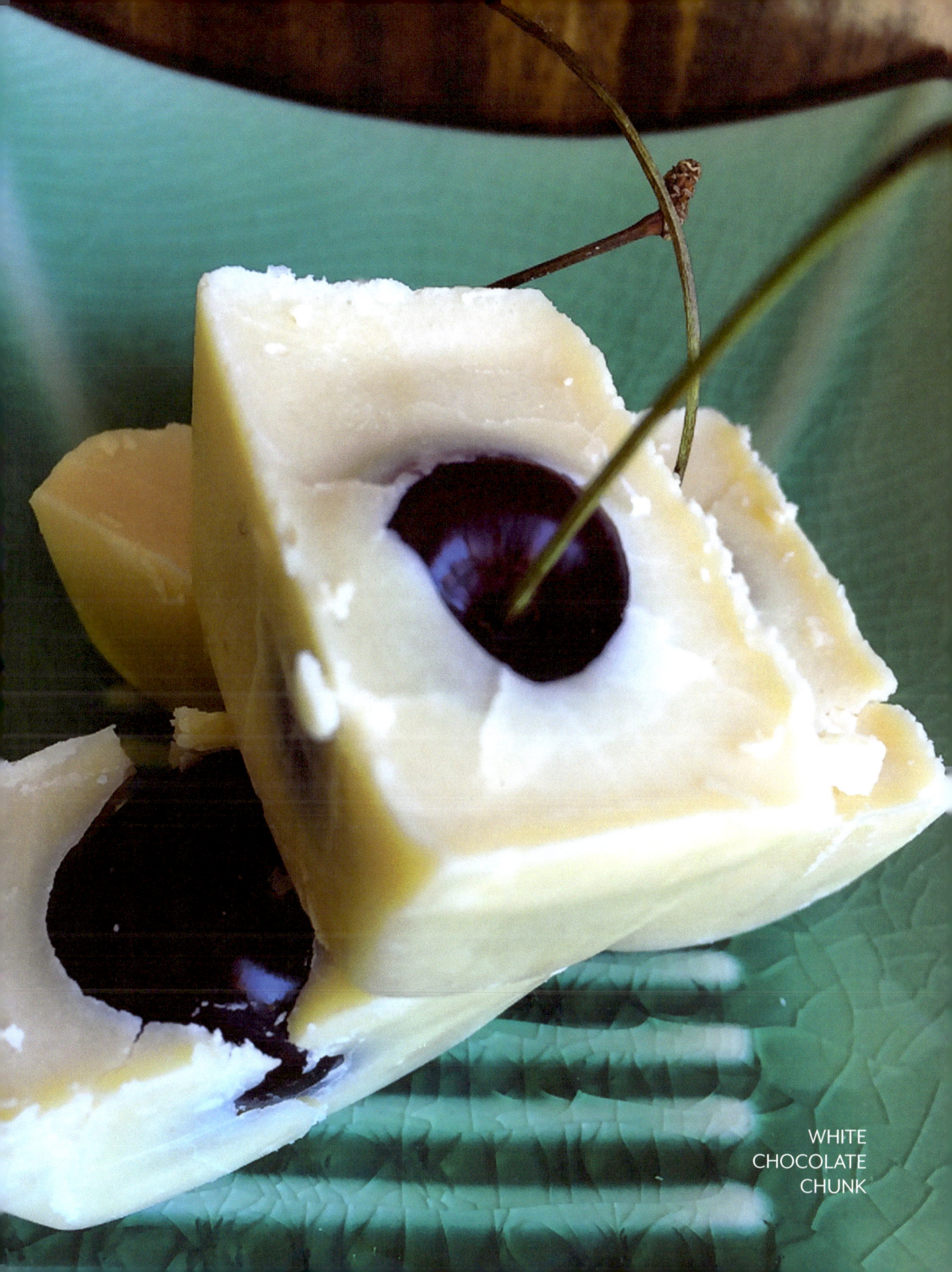

WHITE CHOCOLATE CHUNK

The Chocolate Road

White and dark chocolate combine to make this decidedly smooth road for raw vegans and chocolate lovers everywhere.

A resurfaced road? Yes, there may have been some bumps and rocks along life's path, but now it's been smoothed over with some deliciously rich dark chocolate. As it should be! It's a fitting metaphor. Often the bumps in our life can be soothed with a little chocolate.

This one is dairy free and free from refined sugar. By using maple syrup and stevia for the sweetness, the fructose is kept at a minimum. The result is a silky smooth melt-in-your-mouth chocolate that is rich, delicious but not as addictive as the commercial kind.

Feel free to halve the recipe if you'd like to start with a smaller batch. It will work just as well. You may also want to omit the raspberries and replace them with some almonds and dried sultanas.

INGREDIENTS

White Chocolate

- 1 cup cacao butter (melted)
- 1/2 cup cashews (soaked in water for a few hours or overnight)
- 1/3 cup pure maple syrup
- 1 tbs vanilla extract
- 1 cup raspberries (optional)

Dark Chocolate

- 1 cup coconut oil
- 3/4 cup cacao powder
- 1/4 cup maple syrup
- 1 tbs vanilla extract
- a crackle of pink salt on top

METHOD

White Chocolate

Mix all ingredients in a food processor until smooth. Pour into a square tin lined with baking paper. Top with 1 cup of raspberries then refrigerate. Make the dark chocolate layer.

Dark Chocolate

Blend all ingredients in the food processor. (No need to wash after making the white chocolate.) Pour over the raspberries and refrigerate. Top with a fine crackle of pink salt. Slice into small pieces as it is super rich.

Boost the sweetness with vanilla stevia drops. Enhance the white chocolate flavor with Medicine Flower white chocolate drops.

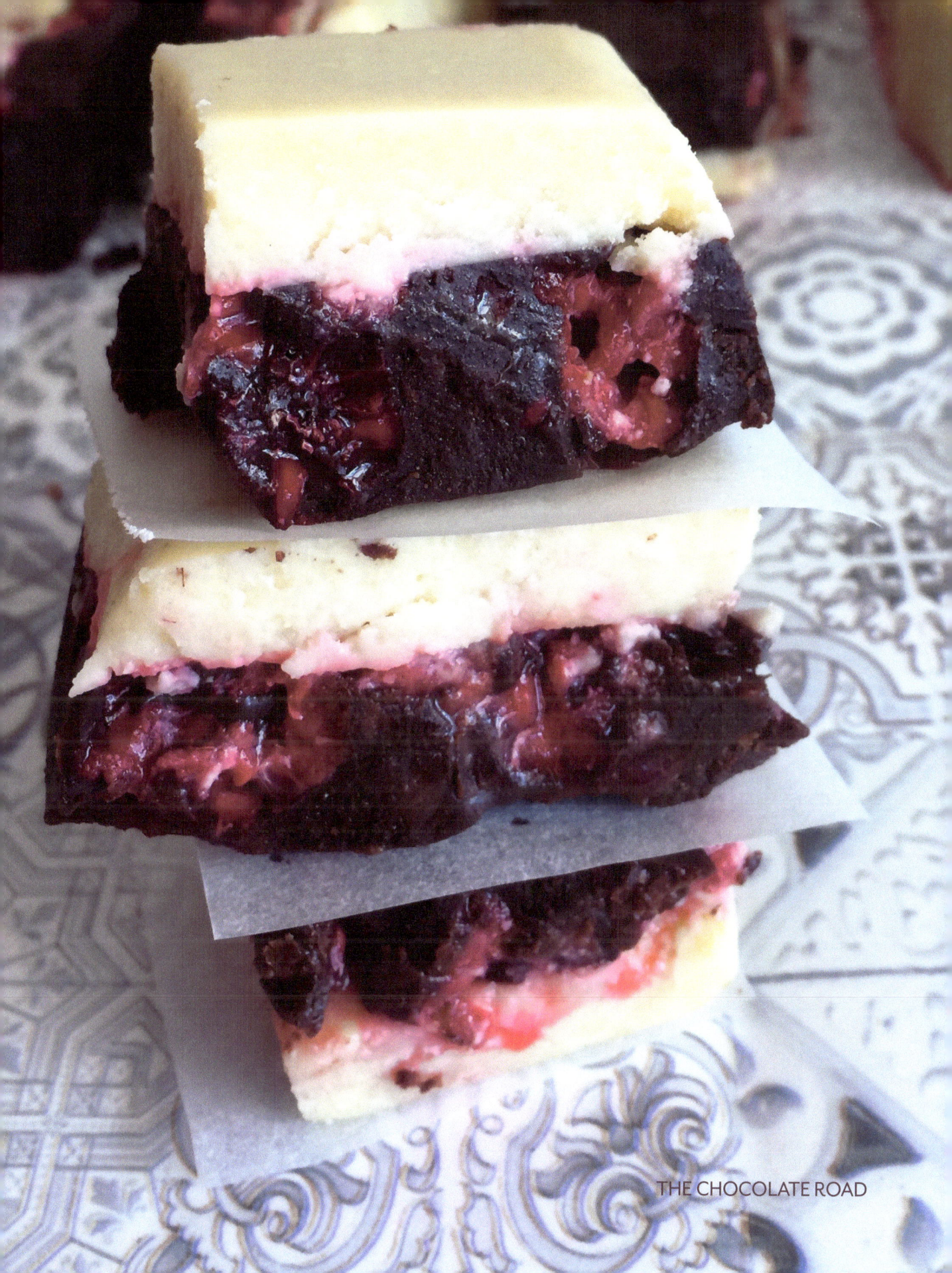
THE CHOCOLATE ROAD

Chocolate Peppermint Slice

INGREDIENTS

Base

- 2 cups almonds (or almond pulp)
- 1/2 cup desiccated coconut
- 1/2 cup xylitol
- 1/2 cup cacao powder
- 1/2 cup cacao butter (could substitute with coconut oil)
- crackle of the salt grinder

Chocolate Peppermint Layer

- 1 1/2 cups cashews (soaked for several hours)
- 3/4 cup cacao powder
- 3/4 cup coconut oil
- 1 cup rice malt syrup
- 10 – 20 drops pure peppermint essence
- crackle of salt grinder

White Choc Mint Layer

- 1 1/2 cups cashews (soaked for several hours)
- 1 cup rice malt syrup
- 1/3 cup cacao butter
- 1/4 cup coconut oil
- 10 -20 drops pure peppermint oil

METHOD

Base

Blend all ingredients in a food processor. Press into a large square tin lined with baking paper.

Chocolate Peppermint Layer

Blend all ingredients until smooth. Add the peppermint essence a drop at a time until you reach your desired flavor. I used 20 drops. Blend, then pour onto the base and freeze

White Choc Mint Layer

Blend all ingredients in food processor until smooth and creamy. Pour onto dark chocolate layer and then allow to set for several hours in the fridge or freezer. Serving suggestion: Top with some raw chocolate sauce and swirl with a knife, or reserve a little of the chocolate layer to swirl on top.

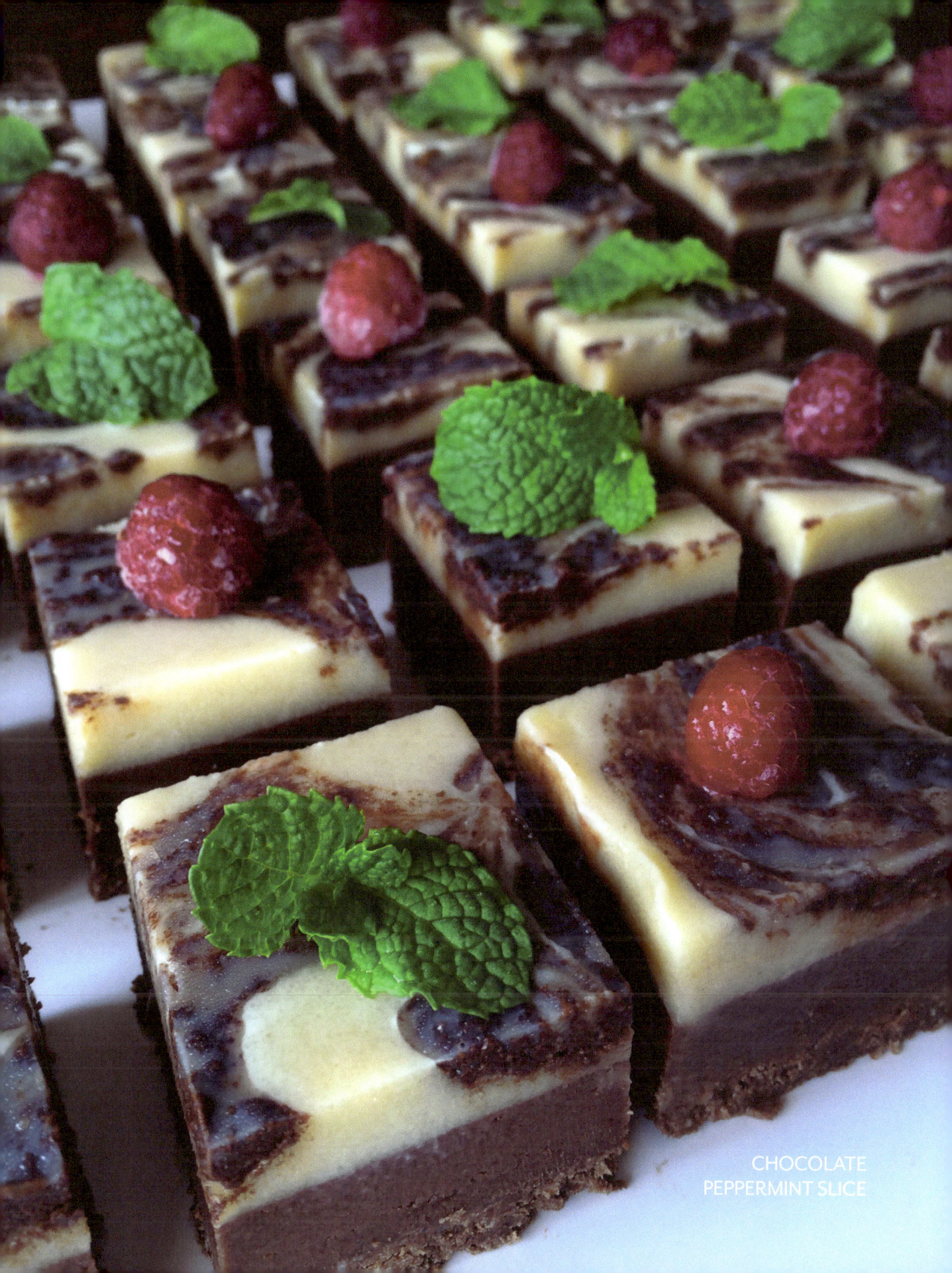

CHOCOLATE PEPPERMINT SLICE

Maple Walnut Fudge

Fudge is normally made out of cream and sugar, so it's going to astound you just how authentic this clean version tastes. The recipe makes a small batch but can quite easily be doubled. I recommend using the small bowl on your food processor. Make sure you use 100% pure maple syrup.

INGREDIENTS

- 1/2 cup coconut paste
- 1/2 cup maple syrup
- 1/4 cup soaked cashews
- 1 tsp vanilla extract (use the kind that has real vanilla seeds)
- 2 tbs walnuts to garnish

METHOD

Blend all ingredients (except walnuts) in a high-powered food processor until creamy and smooth. Pour into a small rectangle tin lined with baking paper and press in some walnuts. Refrigerate or freeze until set. Hmmm, I wish I has some right now.

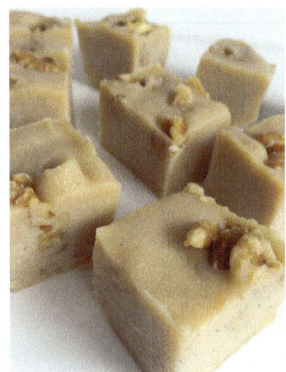
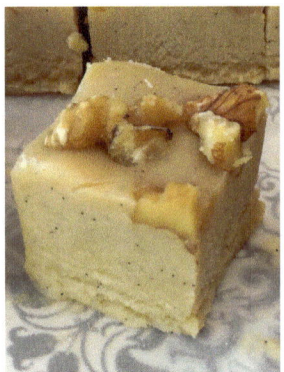

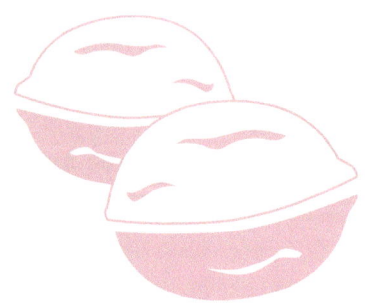

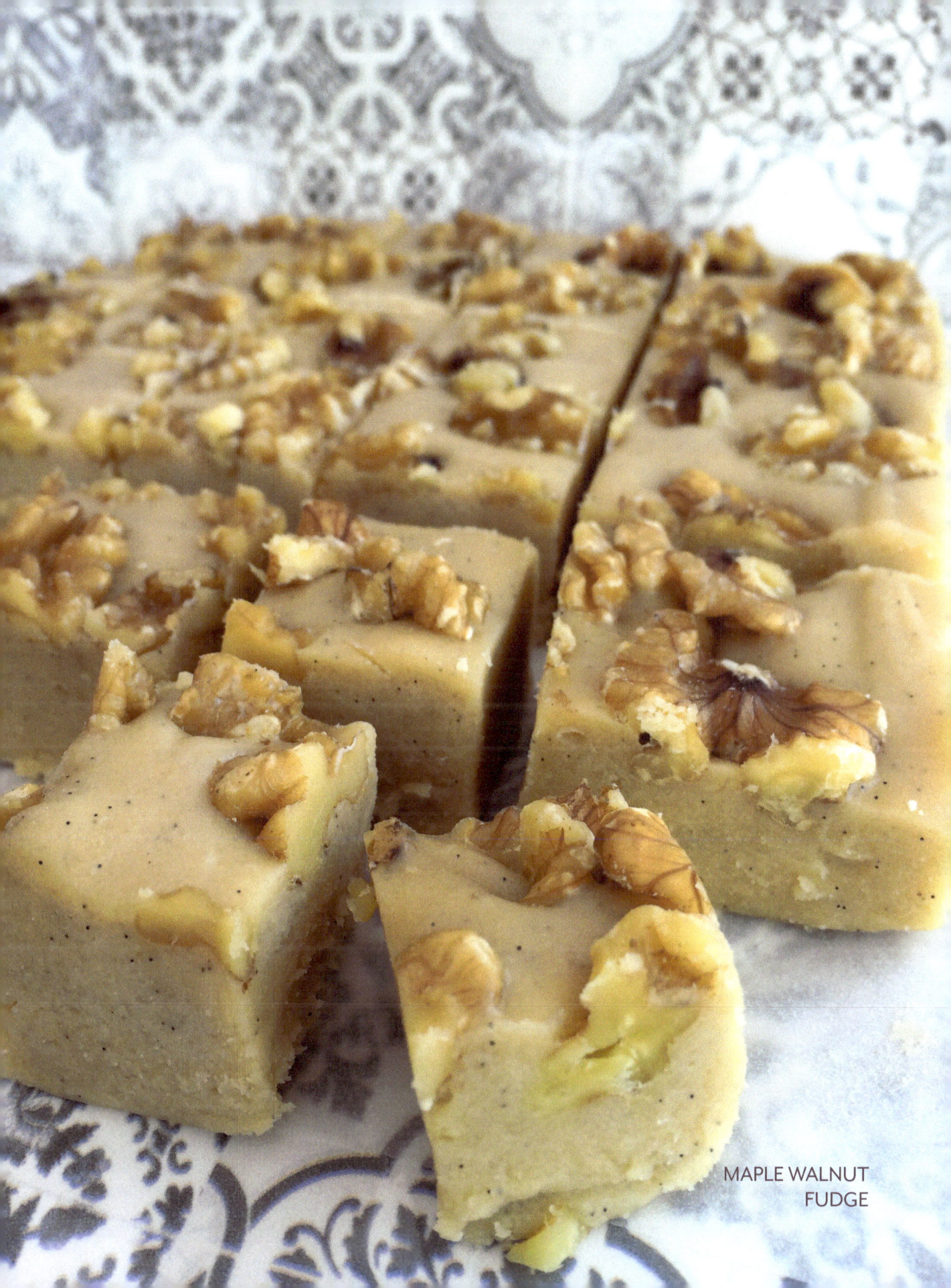

MAPLE WALNUT FUDGE

Chocolate Fudge

Here is the moral dilemma: Easter is just around the corner with all its tempting treats, yet you've just convinced yourself that a detox is a good idea. How about meeting half way? Sipping on your lemon water while those around you munch out on chocolate could make you feel like you've joined the nunnery or some austere group. Try this healthy fudge. Flavor it with orange, a liqueur, or keep it plain. The choices are endless.

INGREDIENTS

- 1/2 cup coconut paste
- 1/4 cup cashews (measure then soak)
- 1/4 cup raw cacao
- 1/2 - 2/3 cup maple syrup (taste as you go)
- 1 tbs vanilla pure essence or extract
- sweet orange essence (5 drops) or zest 1/2 an orange

METHOD

Blend in small food processor until smooth.

Pour into a small tin lined with baking paper and refrigerate.

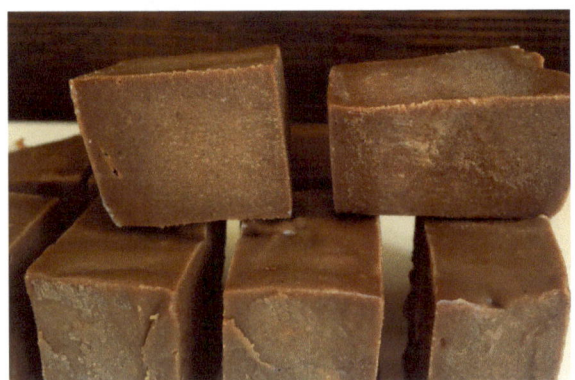

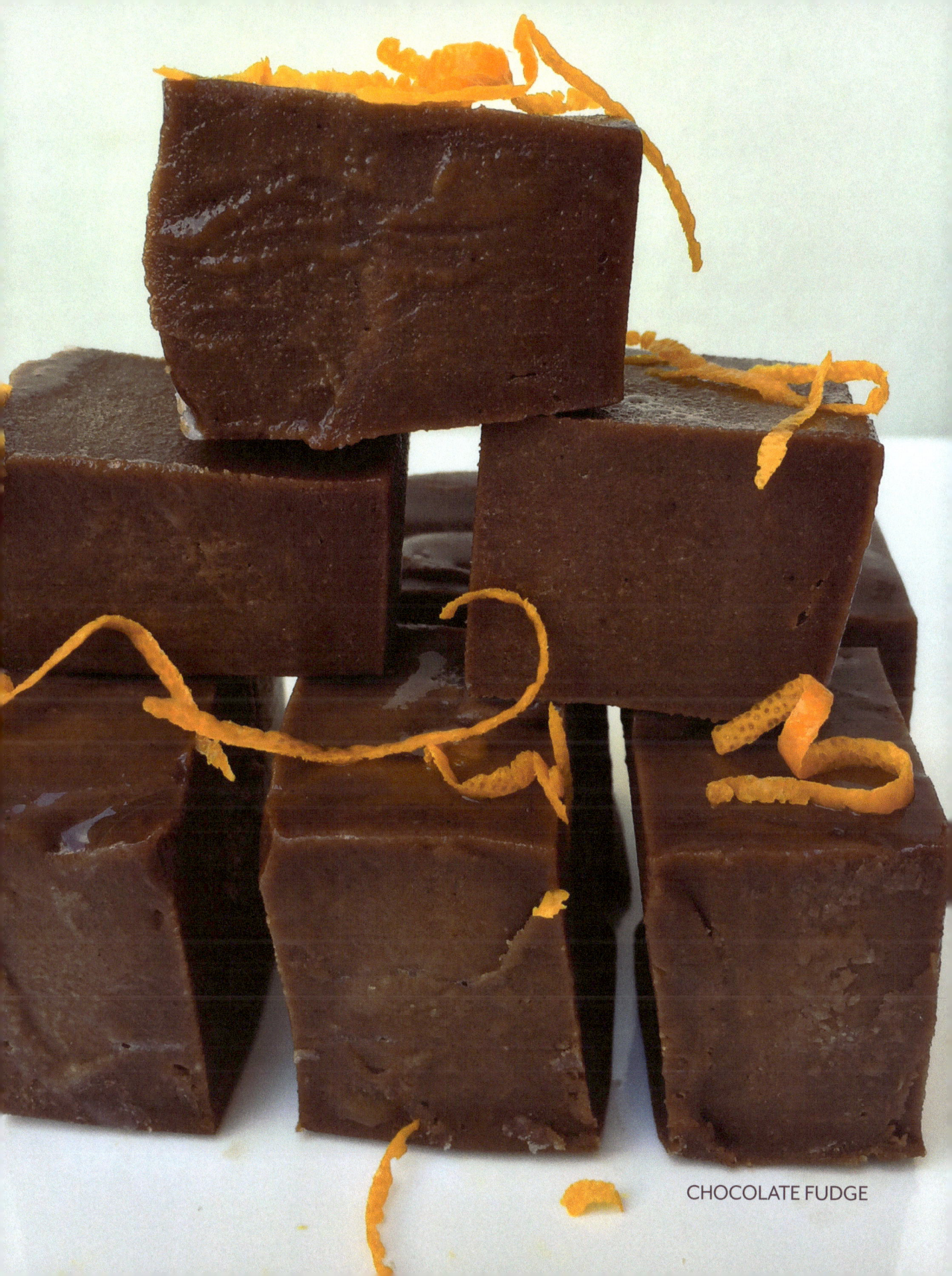

CHOCOLATE FUDGE

Banana Almond Choc Coated Fudge

It's all about the banana fudge. Make this in little fudge filled cups or layer the fudge thickly as a slice (pictured on page 72). Almond butter can be obtained from most health food stores, but be warned; once discovered, many people say it becomes their addiction. They eat it straight from the jar.

INGREDIENTS

Chocolate layer

- 1 cup cacao powder
- 1/2 cup coconut oil
- 1/2 cup cacao butter
- 1/2 cup rice malt syrup
- 1 tbs vanilla extract
- a crackle of salt from the grinder

Banana Fudge Layer

- 1 1/4 cups of almond butter
- 1/2 cup coconut paste
- 1/4 cup coconut oil melted
- 1/4 cup rice malt syrup
- 1/4 cup honey or maple syrup
- 2 bananas
- 1/2 tsp Himalayan salt

METHOD

Chocolate layer

Melt the oil and butter, then combine all ingredients in a bowl or food processor and mix until smooth and glossy. Pour half the mixture into a loaf pan or a small lamington tray. Reserve the other half for the top. Refrigerate until set, then make the fudge.

Banana Fudge Layer

Blend all ingredients in a food processor until very smooth. Spread on to the top of the set chocolate and then pour on the remaining chocolate sauce. Return to the fridge to set. Slice by turning on its side so as not to squash out the fudge or crack the chocolate.

NOTE:

This recipe uses honey for the flavor as well as sweetness. For a vegan or fructose-free alternative, substitute the honey for maple syrup.

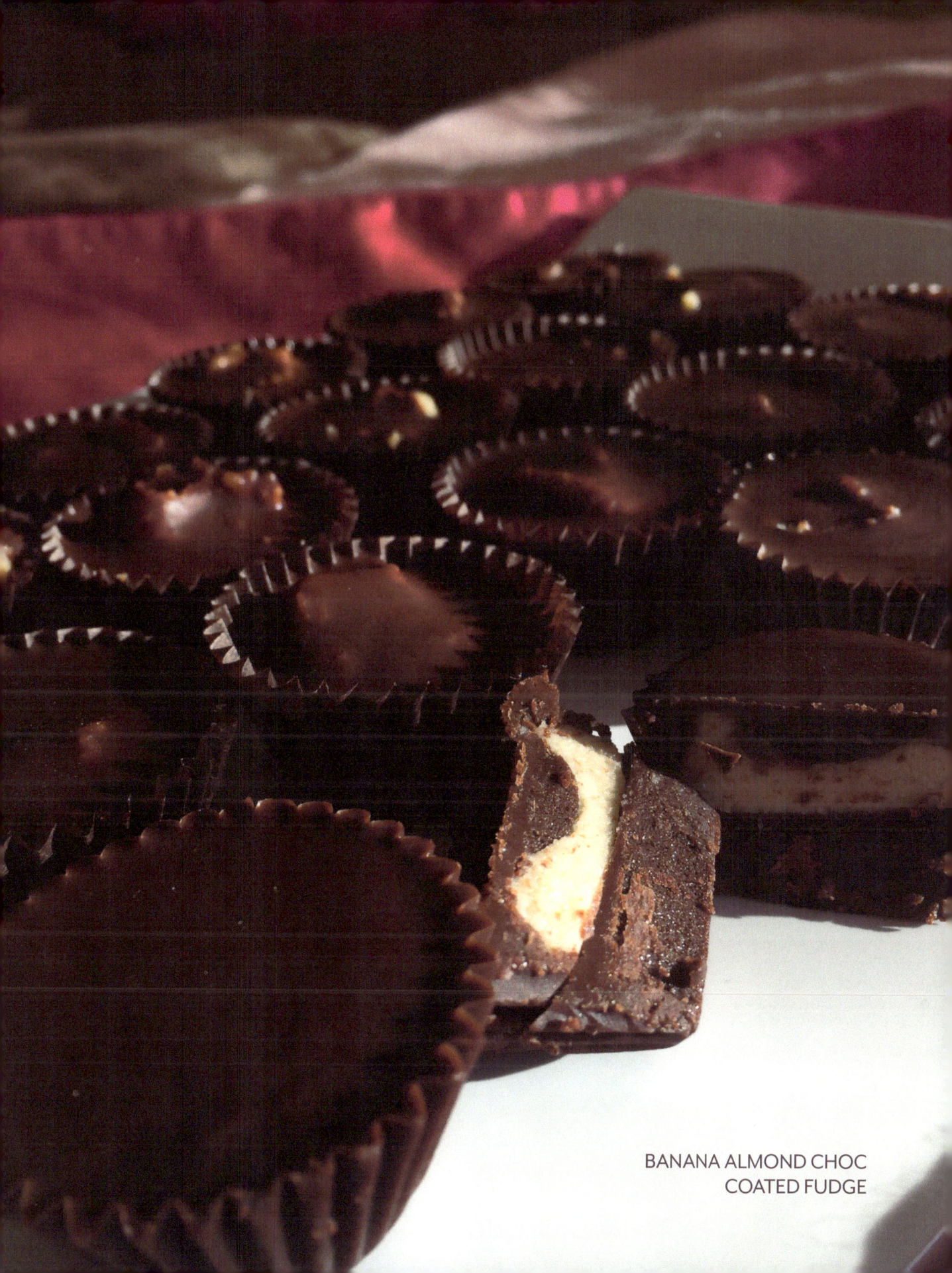

BANANA ALMOND CHOC COATED FUDGE

Chocolate Mousse Parfait

INGREDIENTS

Exotic Chocolate Mousse

- » 1/2 cup melted cacao butter (100g)
- » 1/2 cup raw cacao powder
- » 1/2 cup pure maple syrup
- » 5 white chocolate essence drops (optional)
- » 2 dried apricots + 1 Medjool date + 2 tsp pistachio nuts (to press into the choc discs)
- » 2 cups full fat coconut cream.
- » 2 tsp vanilla extract + 1tbs maple syrup

Draw circles onto the baking paper as a template. Use the top of the parfait glass and make the discs slightly bigger so that the chocolate will form a lid.

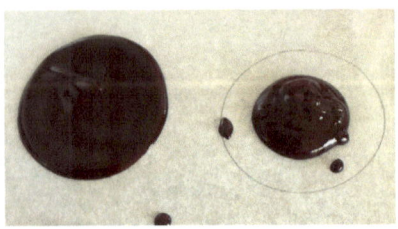

METHOD

Exotic Chocolate Mousse

First make the chocolate discs.

Mix cacao butter, cacao powder, maple syrup and essence in a small glass jug or bowl until smooth and glossy. Draw four circles on baking paper by tracing around the top of the serving glass or parfait glass. Spoon a dollop of chocolate onto the drawn circle and spread into a chocolate disc. Repeat with the remaining 3 circles. Reserve the remaining chocolate for the mousse. Press into the chocolate slices of dried apricot, Medjool dates and pistachio nuts. Refrigerate.

Chocolate Mousse

Whip 1 cup coconut cream with the remaining chocolate sauce. (There should be about 2/3 cup left. Pour into a piping bag or use a sandwich bag inserted in a glass. Refrigerate until it firms up.

Vanilla Cream

Whip the remaining 1 cup of coconut cream with 1 tsp vanilla paste and 1 tbs maple syrup. Pour into a piping bag and refrigerate until firm.

Serve this dairy free mousse in your favorite parfait glasses.

If using a sandwich bag instead of a piping bag, snip a small corner off the plastic. Keep an even pressure on the bag and pipe chocolate and vanilla mousse into glasses in alternate layers. Two of each should do. Peel off chocolate discs from the baking paper and place on top of glasses.

Serve with peppermint tea and fresh berries.

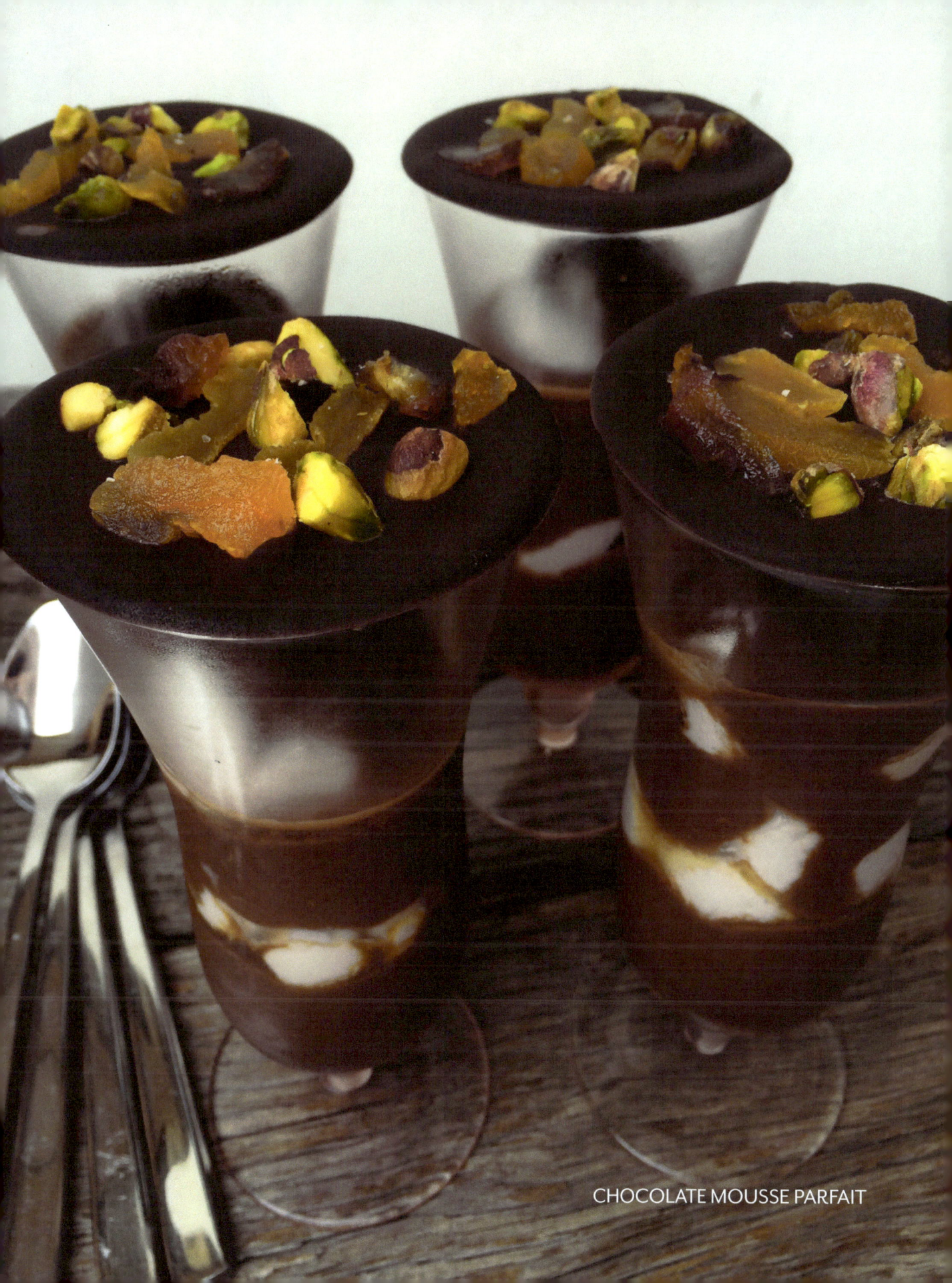

CHOCOLATE MOUSSE PARFAIT

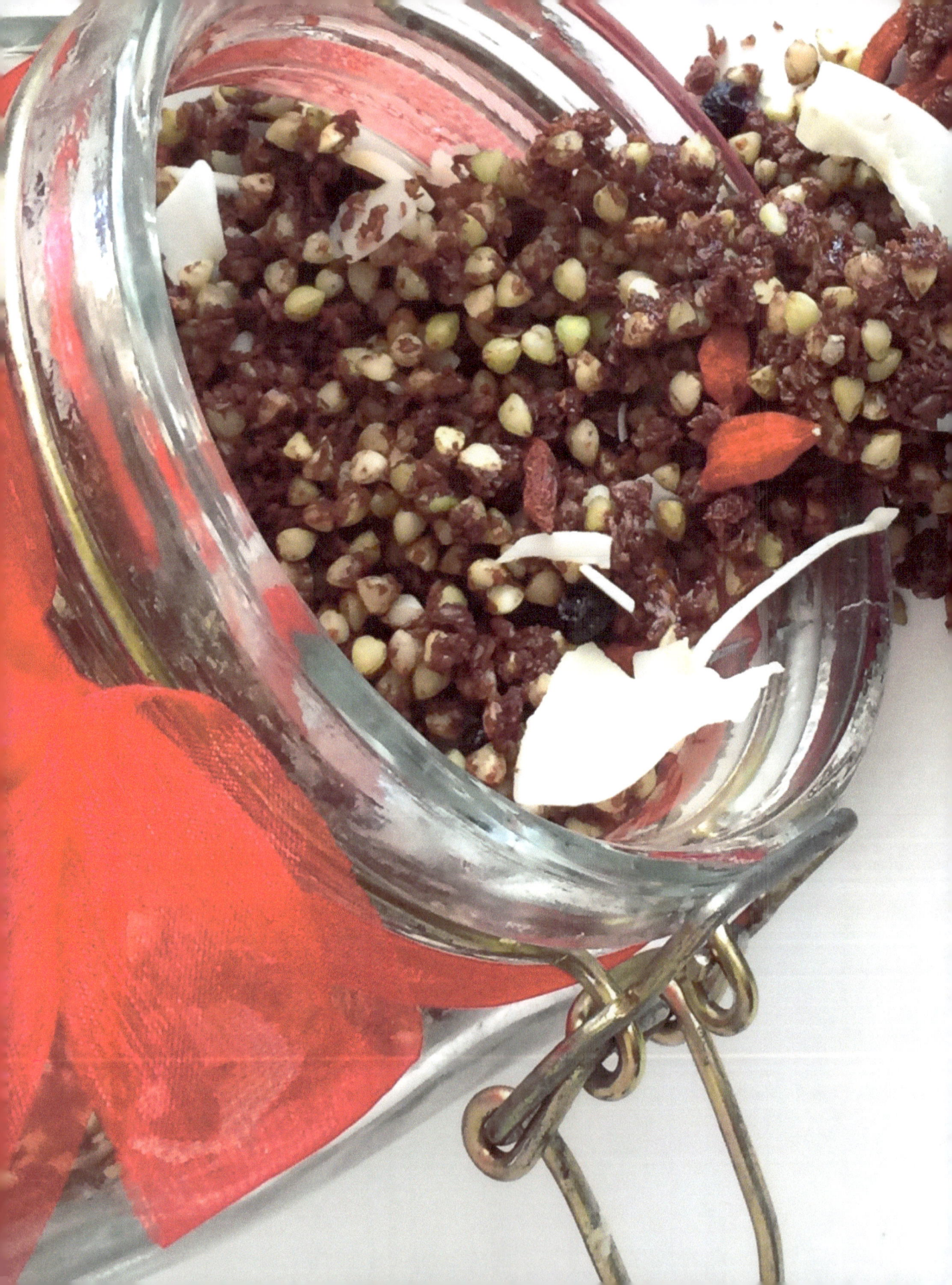

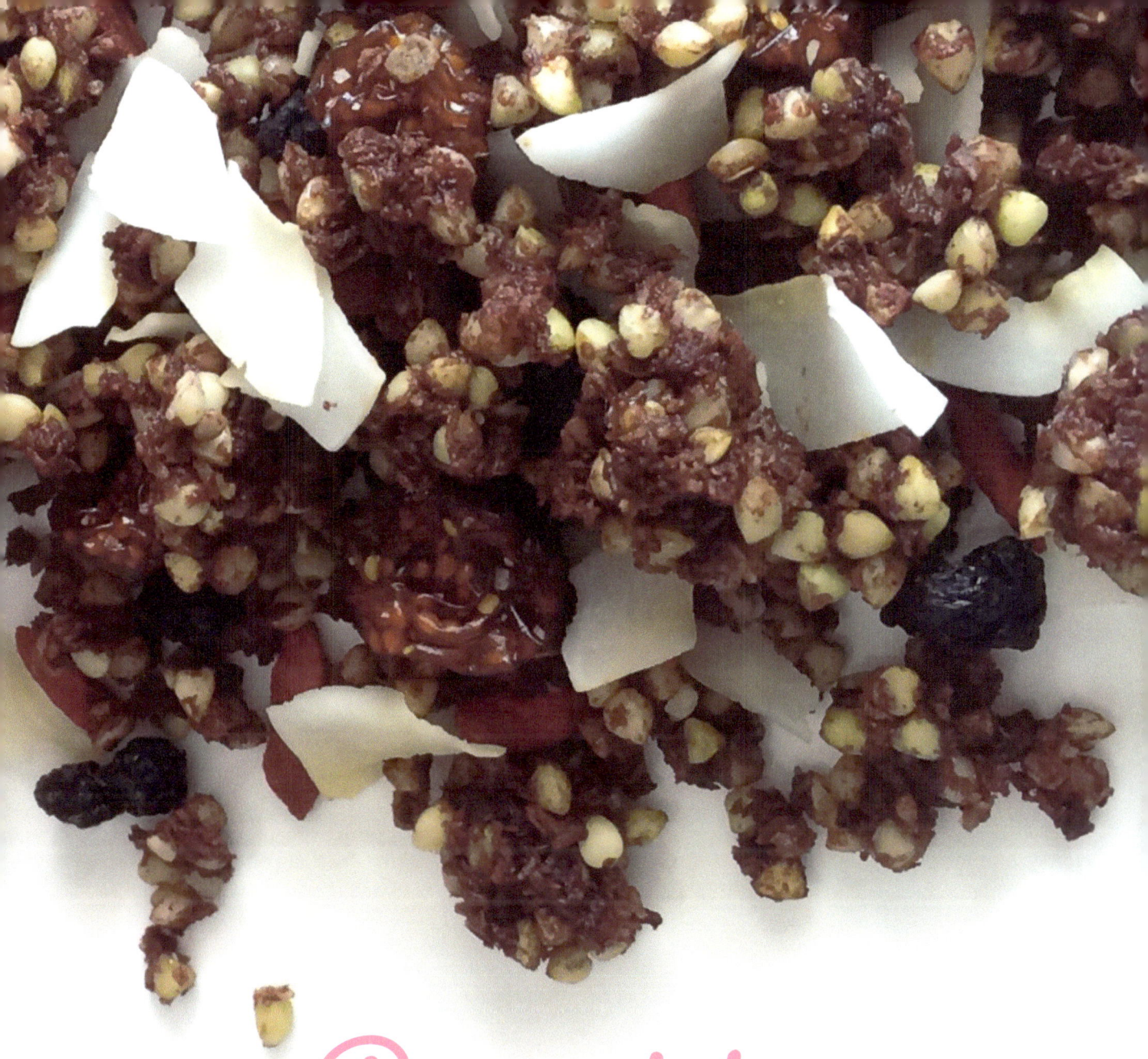

Breakfast Desserts

Blueberry Pikelets

These might as well be called brain enhancing, youth regenerating little circles of yummy goodness. Blueberries are well known for their high antioxidant properties and flaxseed is a fabulous vegan source of omega 3s, which are known to improve brain function. Did you know that flaxseed is also called linseed? Be sure to use the left over almond pulp from your homemade almond milk.

INGREDIENTS

- 1 cup almond meal
- 1/2 cup linseeds
- 2 tbs chia seeds
- 1/4 cup rice malt syrup
- 1/2 cup freshly squeezed orange juice
- 1/4 cup desiccated coconut
- 1 cup of blueberries
- Maple syrup to serve

METHOD

Crack the linseeds in a 1 second blitz using a spice grinder. This means just break open their shell so that some might still be whole and some are a little ground. In a bowl, mix the almond meal, chia seeds, linseeds, syrup, juice and coconut until well combined into a dough. Add the blueberries, being careful not to squash them.

Make little round balls from the dough and press them onto a lined piece of baking paper. Dehydrate for one hour and then flip to dry for a further hour. Serve warm with maple syrup and coconut yoghurt or just as they are.

Dehydrate these for longer to turn them into cookies with a longer shelf life.

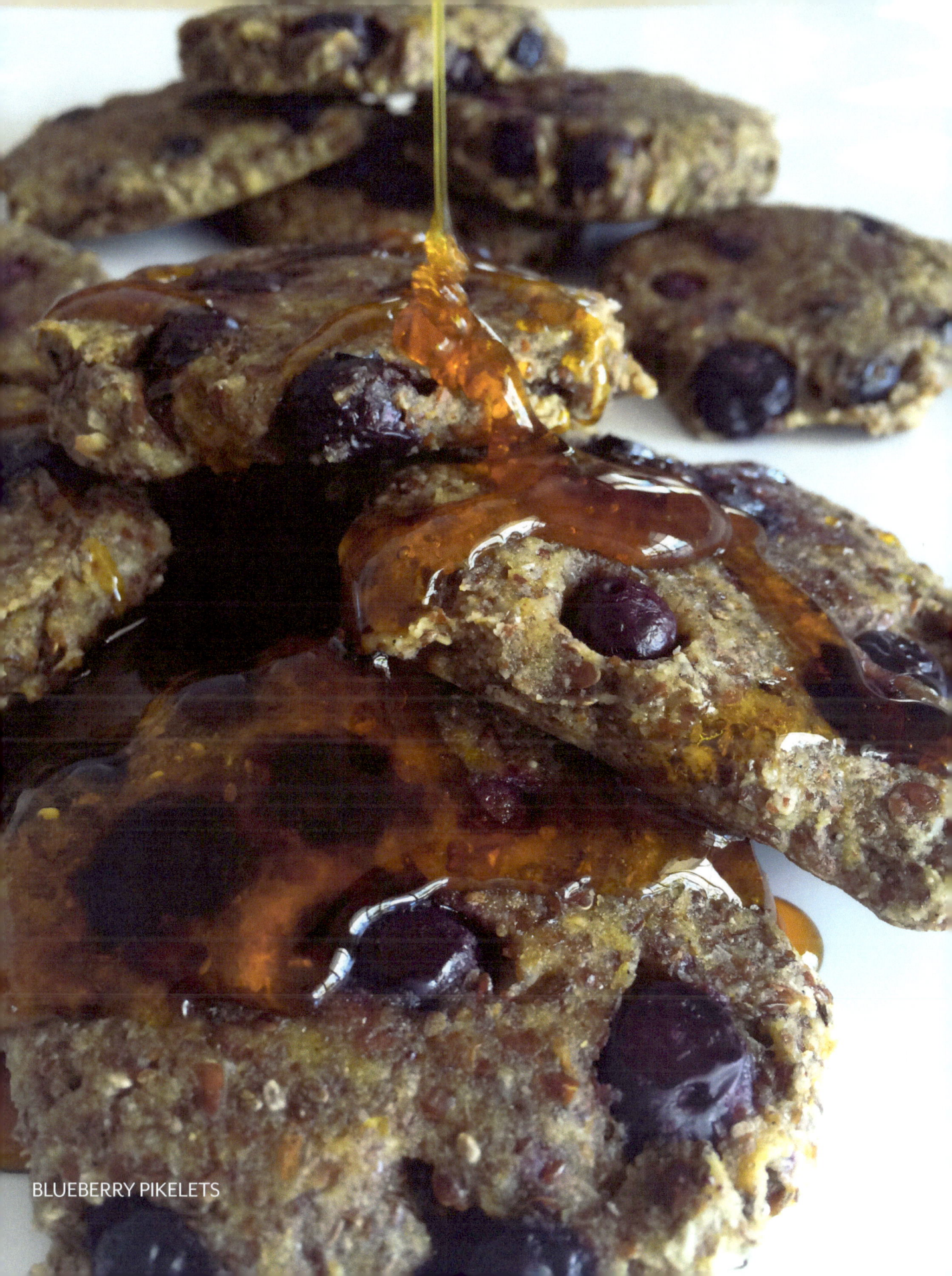

BLUEBERRY PIKELETS

Chocolate Buckini Muesli with Almond Milk

Raw means refined cereals such as cocoa pops and milk are off the menu. But don't for a moment think that you have to be deprived of chocolatey breakfast type cereals forever. Try this homemade granola made with buckwheat.

It's easy to think that buckwheat is another grain. No, it is not even related to wheat. Buckwheat is a tasty fruit seed with a host of immune boosting minerals. Manganese, magnesium, copper, and zinc are just some of its treasures. It also contains all eight essential amino acids, including lysine. Kiss cold sores good-bye with this breakfast cereal.

INGREDIENTS

- 1 heaped cup buckwheat (soaked for several hours) or use buckinis
- 1/4 cup raw cacao powder
- 1/2 cup desiccated coconut
- 1/4 cup xylitol
- 2 tbs coconut oil
- 2 tbs water if you have used dry buckinis
- 1 cup mixed dried super fruits such as goji berries, cranberries, currants etc.

METHOD

Mix all ingredients together until well combined. Spread on a baking tray or dehydrator sheets and allow to dehydrate. Or eat immediately with homemade vanilla almond milk. See recipe for almond milk in 'The Basics'.

NOTE:

I added the oil and water because I wanted the mix to clump together into chunky chocolatey morsels. You could omit these two ingredients and skip the drying time, but only if you have used dry buckinis in the first place. The mix needs to be dry to store in the pantry.

To save time, you can buy buckwheat that has already been activated and then dehydrated (buckinis).

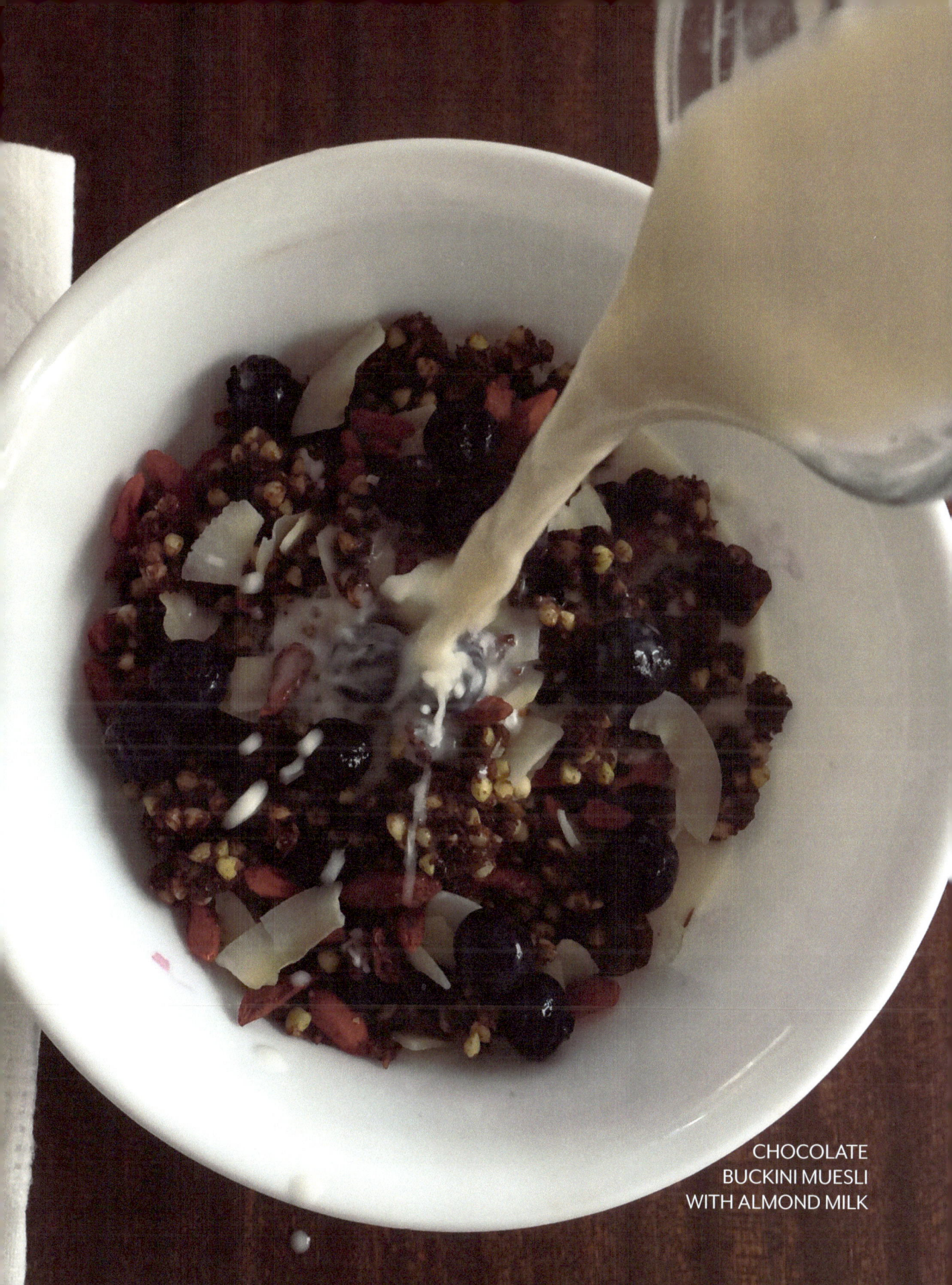

CHOCOLATE
BUCKINI MUESLI
WITH ALMOND MILK

Pear and Raspberry Chia Porridge

This is a lovely raw recipe that is great for winter. The use of Brazil nuts makes this particularly nutritious. The benefits of selenium are many:

- Helps promote a healthy liver
- Protects against toxic metals in the body including mercury
- Protects against heart disease
- Neutralizes alcohol, smoke and fats
- Acts as an antioxidant against free radicals
- May help prevent cancers.

Selenium is also important for the healthy function of the thyroid gland because it helps make several thyroid enzymes.

INGREDIENTS

- 1 cup water (hot)
- 1/3 cup chia seeds
- 1/3 cup Brazil nuts
- 1/3 cup coconut cream
- 2 ripe pears (or 1 pear and 1 banana)
- 2/3 cup raspberries
- 1 tbs maple syrup (for garnish)

METHOD

Reserve some pear and berries for garnish, then blend all other ingredients in blender, adding hot water last. Pour into bowls. Top with fresh sliced fruit and a drizzle of maple syrup. Serves two.

If you have used frozen berries, then warm the porridge further on the stove or dehydrator under a low temperature. Brazil nuts can be omitted and replaced with extra coconut cream. But since Brazil nuts are nature's highest source of selenium I'd keep them in.

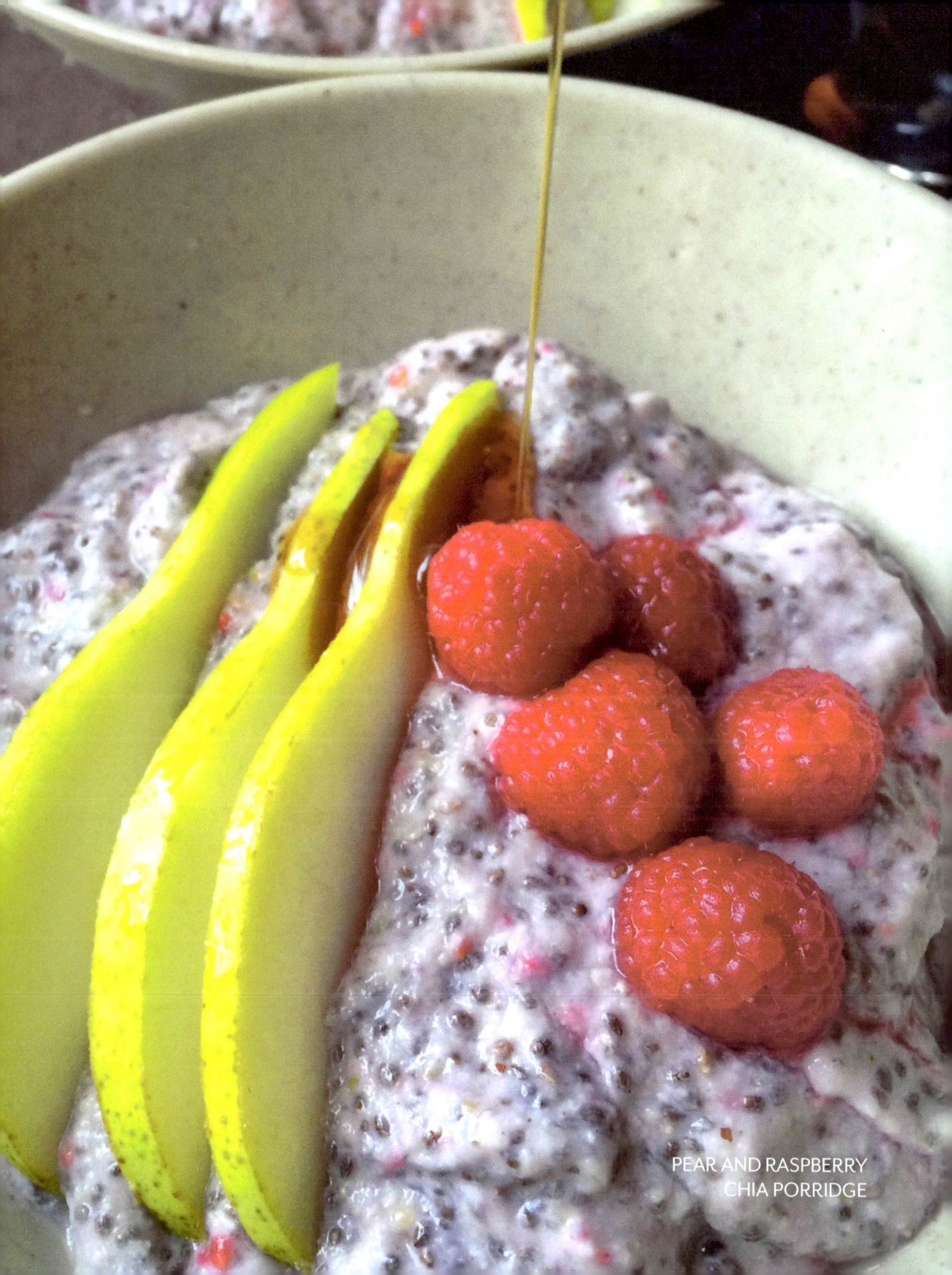

PEAR AND RASPBERRY CHIA PORRIDGE

Strawberry Coconut Chia Pudding

Chia seeds are a good source of protein, high in fiber, low in calories, and contain antioxidant properties. They are also a good vegan source of Omega 3 fatty acids.

Since Chia seeds are virtually tasteless, they are like a blank canvas for whatever you soak them in. Today, soak them in coconut cream for a taste of the tropics.

INGREDIENTS

- 1 cup pure coconut cream
- 1/4 cup chia seeds
- 1 tsp stevia powder or your choice of sweetener (1 tbs maple syrup)
- 1/2 tsp vanilla extract
- 1 cup of strawberries or fruit of your choice (banana or pineapple)

METHOD

Blend chia seeds, coconut cream, vanilla, fruit and stevia in a blender until smooth. Pour into a Mason jar with a lid. Refrigerate for a few hours until set. Allow time for the chia seeds to absorb the liquid. Serve with additional fruit or as is.

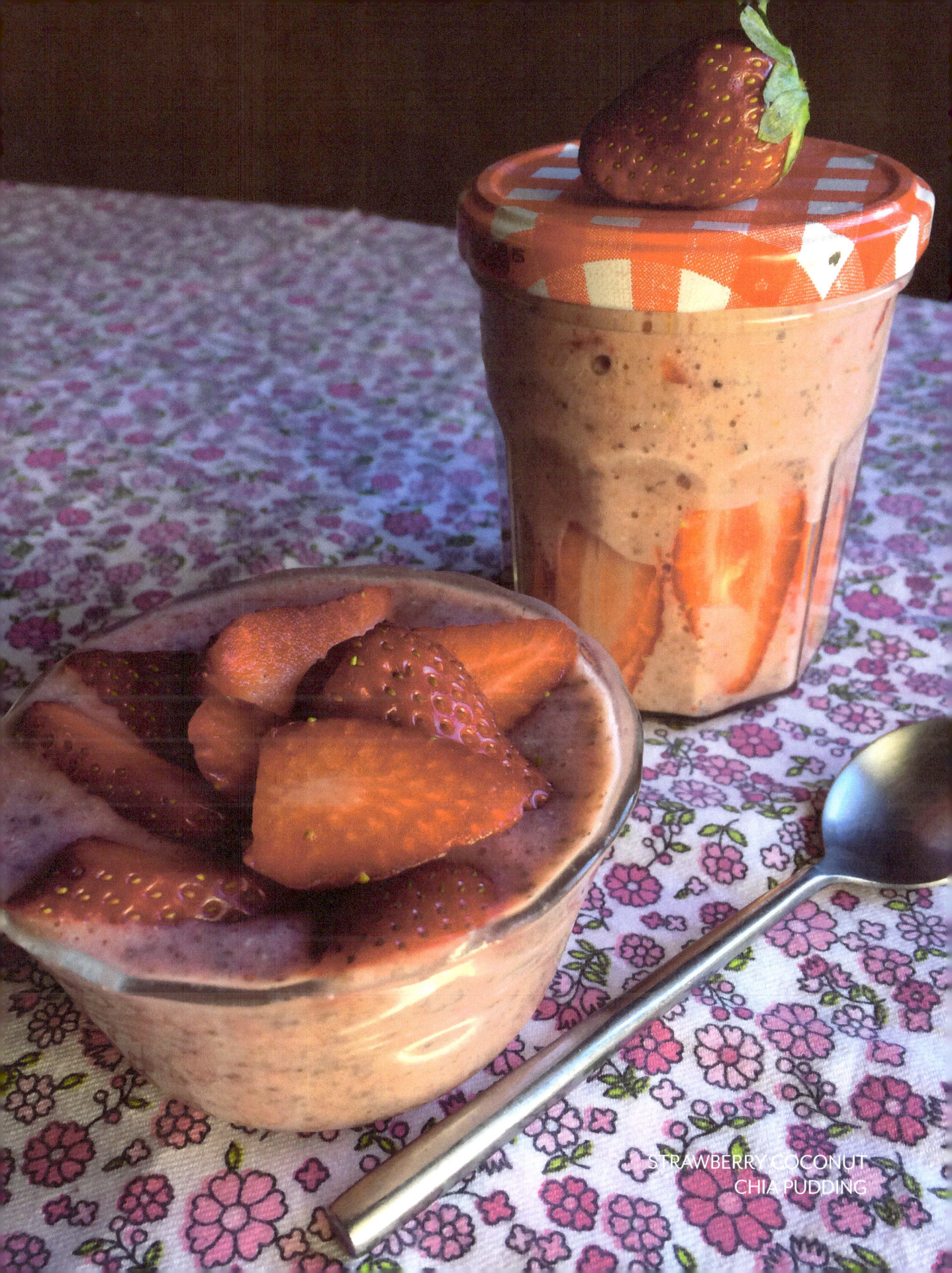

STRAWBERRY COCONUT
CHIA PUDDING

Green Chia Pudding

This recipe is so simple, you'll wonder why you didn't think of it sooner. It's high in protein, good fats for the brain, vitamins and full fiber from the whole fruit. Many people start the day with a freshly squeezed orange juice. This recipe will give your juice a protein boost and slow the release of glucose into the blood.

A breakfast that includes protein leaves you feeling satiated and less likely to snack in between meals. It gives you sustained energy for the day and eaten after a strenuous workout will give you the building blocks to carry out muscle growth and repair.

INGREDIENTS

- 1 orange, freshly squeezed
- 1 banana
- 1/2 an avocado
- 2 tbs chia seeds
- 1-2 tbs water

METHOD

Blend all ingredients in the food processor. Pour into small glasses and set in the fridge for an hour or two. Serves two.

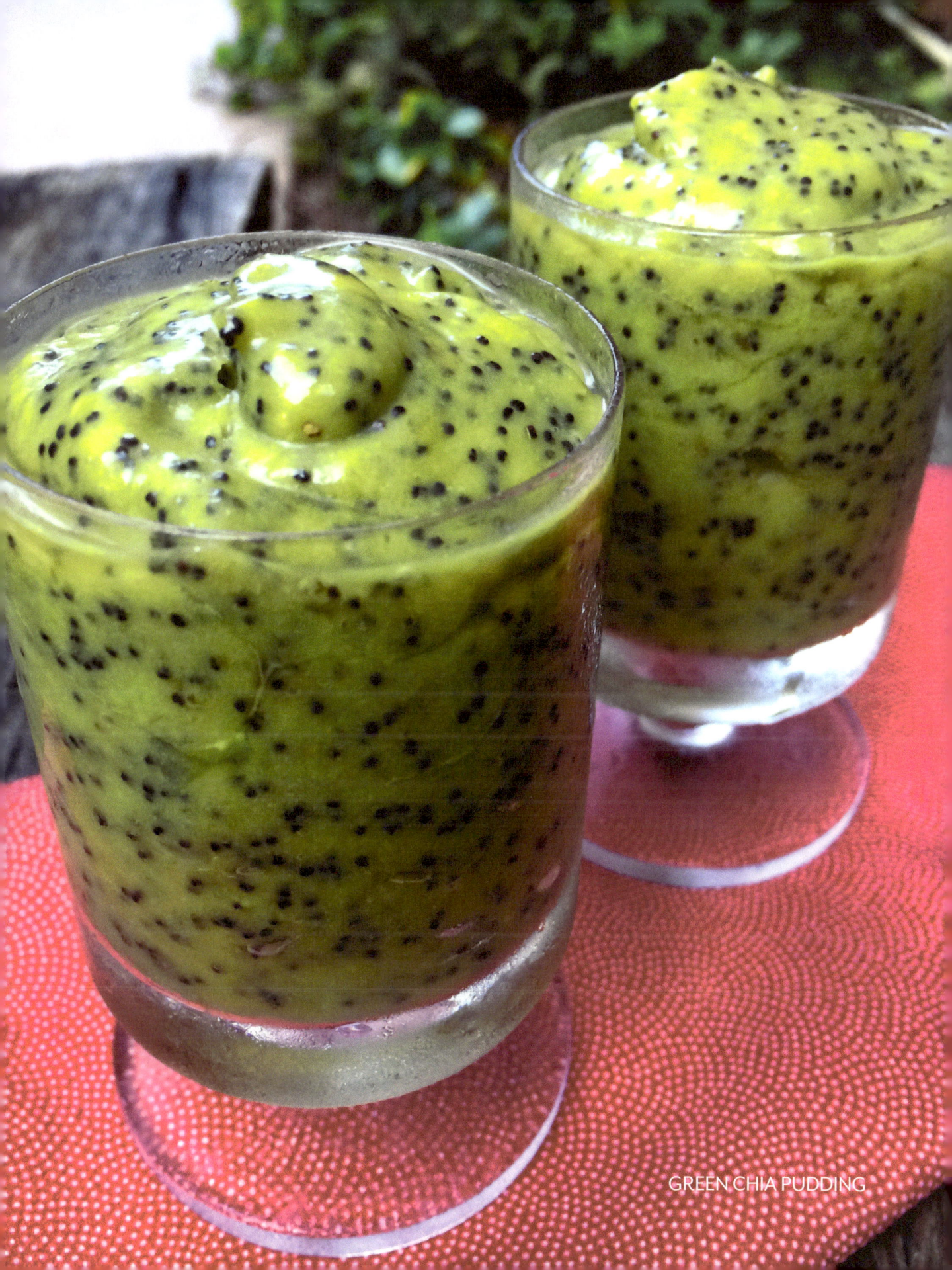
GREEN CHIA PUDDING

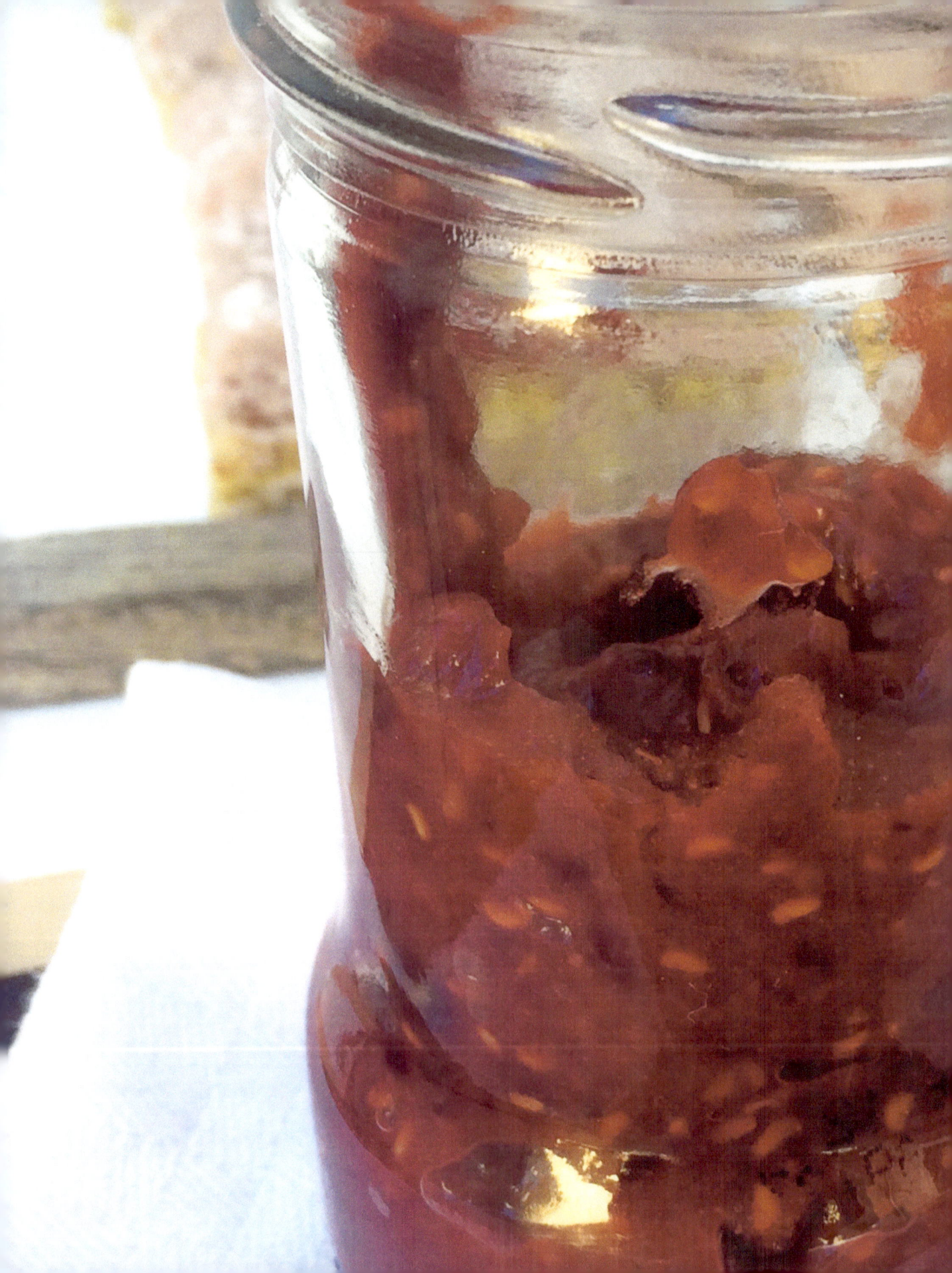

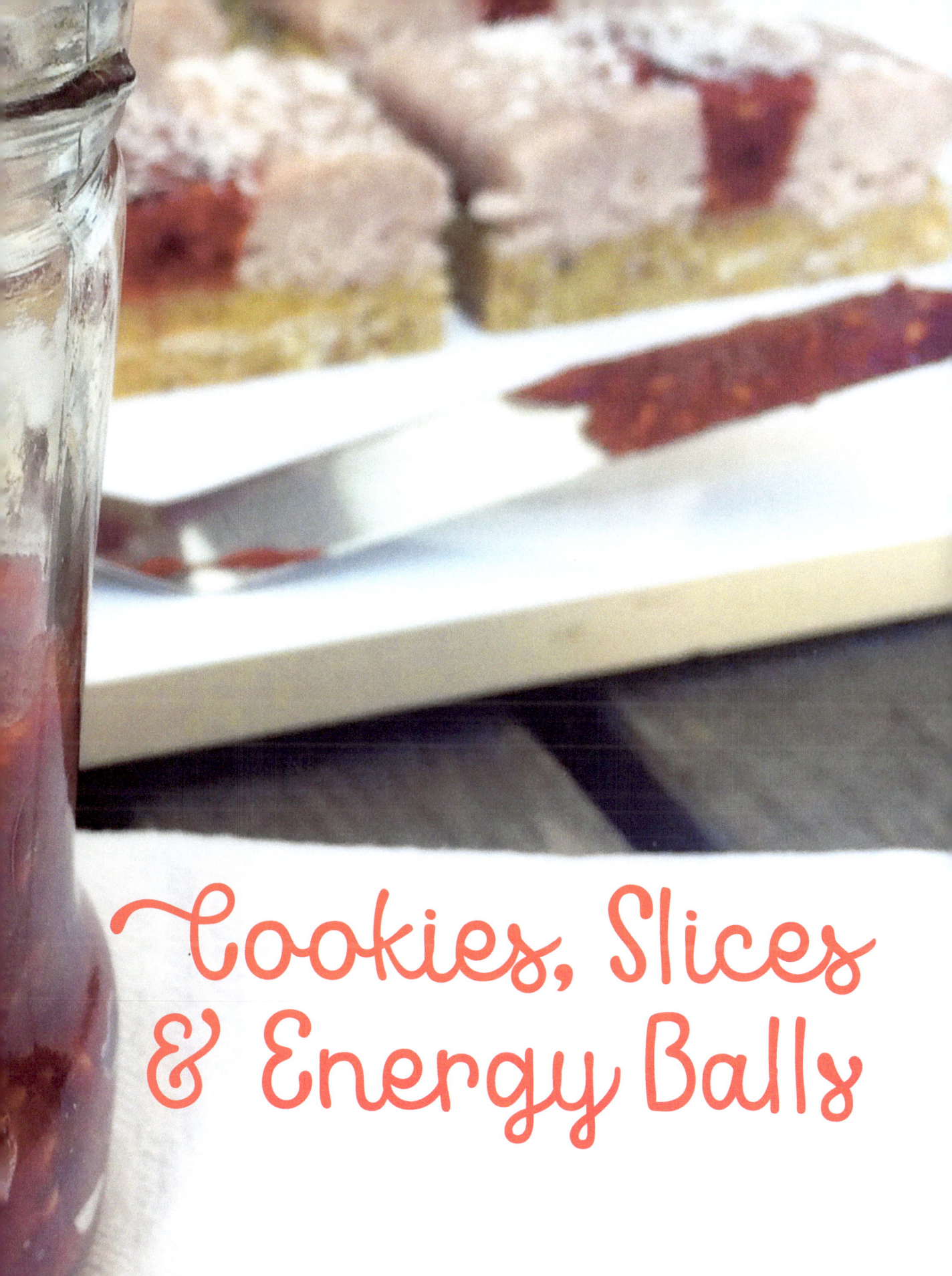

Cookies, Slices & Energy Balls

Banana and Mango Hemp Cookies

What's in a cookie if there is no butter, flour, or eggs?
Let this recipe surprise and satisfy your cookie craving.

INGREDIENTS

- 1 banana
- 2 mangoes
- 1 cup almonds (or use leftover pulp from making almond milk)
- 2 tbs chia seeds
- 1/2 cup hemp seeds (or substitute with raw oats)
- 2 tbs coconut oil
- 1/2 cup desiccated coconut
- 1/2 lime juiced

METHOD

Blend all ingredients in food processor. Dollop spoonfuls onto a baking paper lined tray or silicon sheets. Top with thin slices of banana. Dehydrate in oven or dehydrator below 47 degrees Celcius (110 F) for several hours then flip to continue drying. Keep them chewy. Store in fridge or freezer if not eating within next day.

Makes about 35.

If mangoes aren't in season, then substitute with 250 g of fresh strawberries. You may need to adjust the sweetness with a little stevia because strawberries aren't as sweet as mangoes.

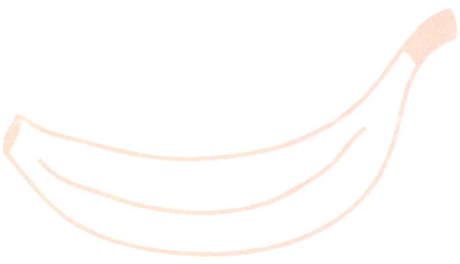

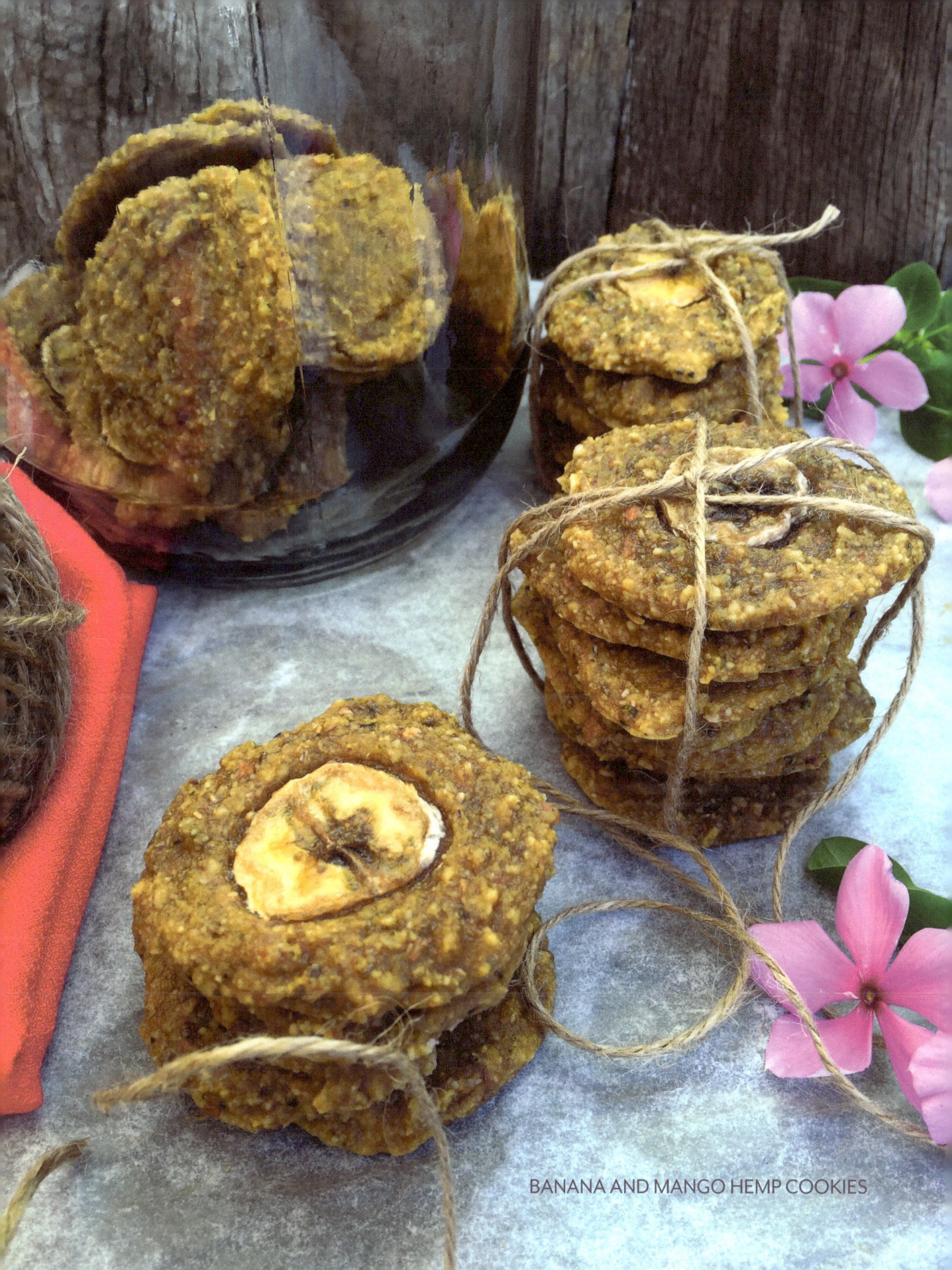

BANANA AND MANGO HEMP COOKIES

Raw Iced VoVo

Arnott's famous Iced VoVo is the inspiration for this biscuit. Yes, it's a healthy Australian cookie recipe! Sticky raspberry jam and chewy coconut? What's not to love? It's like a jam topped macaroon.

I just love taking the naughty out of sweets and desserts because food and eating should be a pleasure, not a guilt-ridden exercise or punishment. When food is used to nourish the body and it tastes spectacular, eating healthily becomes a way of life, not an onerous chore.

INGREDIENTS

Base

- Measure nuts then presoak.
- 1 cup almonds
- 1 cup of cashews
- 1/2 cup coconut flour
- 1/2 cup rice malt syrup
- 1 tsp vanilla extract
- crackle of pink salt

Pink Coconut Layer

- 2 cups desiccated coconut
- 1/2 cup rice malt syrup
- 2 tbs coconut paste (melted)
- 1 2 tbs coconut oil (melted)
- vanilla stevia drops to taste or 1 tsp vanilla extract
- 1 tbs raspberries (for coloring)

Raspberry jam

- 2 cups raspberries
- 3/4 cup pitted dates
- 1/4 cup hot water to soften dates

METHOD

Base

Blend all ingredients in food processor until it forms a ball when squeezed with hand. Press onto a cookie tray lined with baking paper. Use a rolling pin to roll out flat between two pieces of baking paper. Keep it whole; you will slice it later.

Pink Coconut Layer

Blend all ingredients in a food processor. Scrape down sides and blend again for a few minutes until smooth.

Roll pink mixture into sausage lengths or small balls to line the edges of your cookie base. Press onto the base. Leave an empty strip down the middle to fill with raspberry jam. Refrigerate.

Raspberry jam

Pour hot water onto dates in a glass bowl and allow to soften for a few minutes. Blend raspberries and dates in food processor, until dates are broken down. Adjust for sweetness with vanilla stevia drops if you like it sweeter.

Spoon the jam onto the biscuit. Allow to set before slicing into small biscuit-sized portions. Sprinkle with additional coconut to garnish.

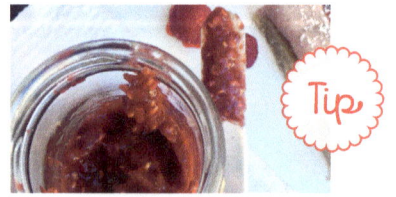

Tip: Be generous when applying this gooey yummy jam.

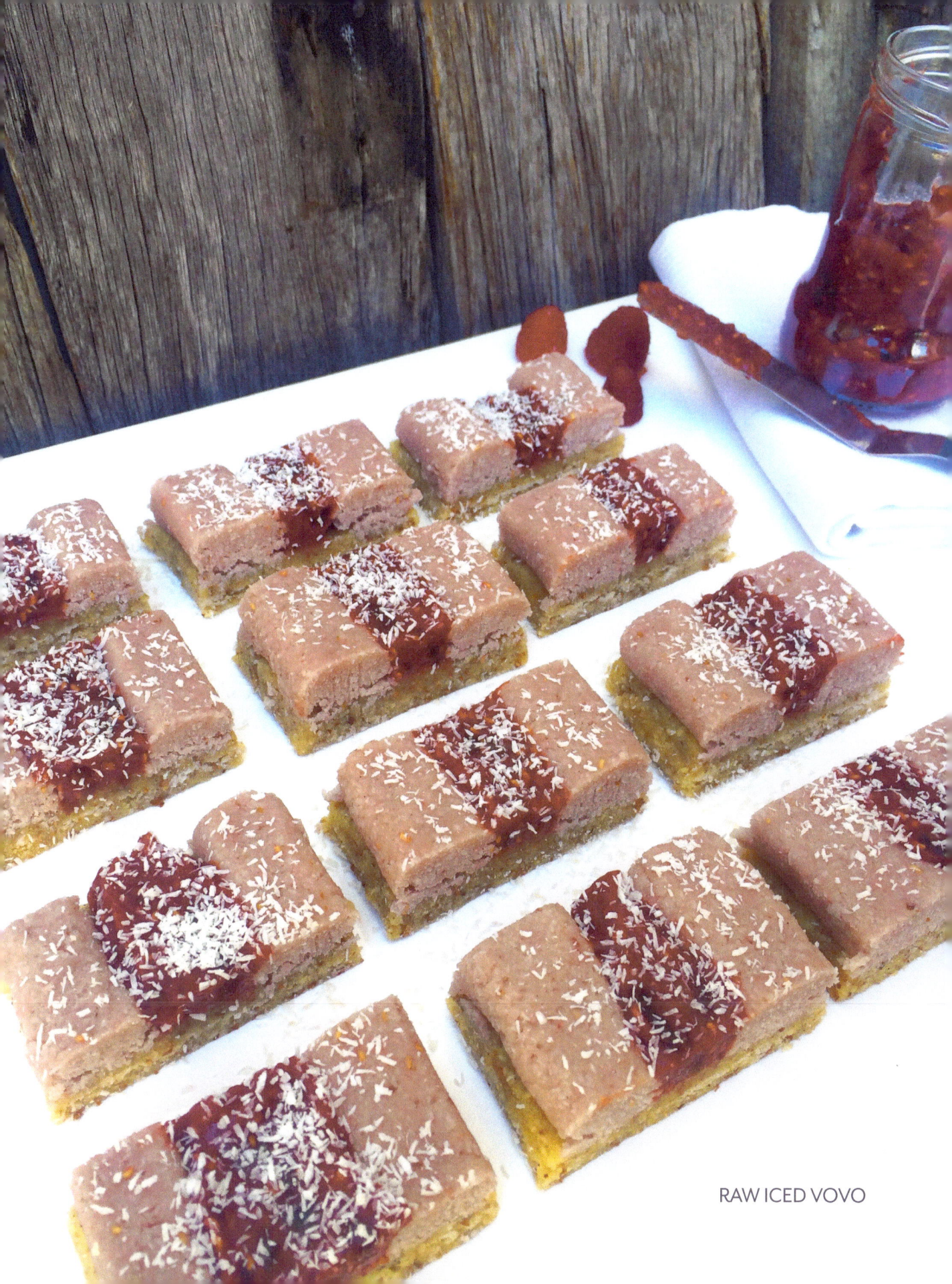
RAW ICED VOVO

Bounty Bar Slice

A retake on the classic Australian chocolate bar.

INGREDIENTS

Base

- 1 cup walnuts
- 1 cup pecans
- 2 tbs cacao powder
- 1 cup sultanas
- 4 Medjool dates
- 2 tbs coconut oil
- 2 tsp vanilla extract or essence
- 1/2 tsp Maldon salt flakes

Coconut layer

- 2 cups desiccated coconut
- 1 cup coconut paste
- 1/2 cup coconut cream
- 1 – 2 tbs vanilla extract
- 2 tbs coconut oil
- 1/2 tsp of salt flakes

METHOD

Base

Blend dry ingredients in food processor until mixture resembles bread crumbs. Add in dried fruit, oil, vanilla and salt. Mix well until a fudgy consistency is reached. Press into a small tin lined with baking paper. Use the back of a spoon to get a smooth finish. Place in fridge to set.

Coconut layer

Blend all ingredients in a food processor. Scrape down sides and blend again until smooth. Pour over the chocolate base and set in the fridge or freezer until firm. Slice into bars.

Tip

If you have any leftover chocolate sauce from one of the other recipes, drizzle it over the top with a spoon.

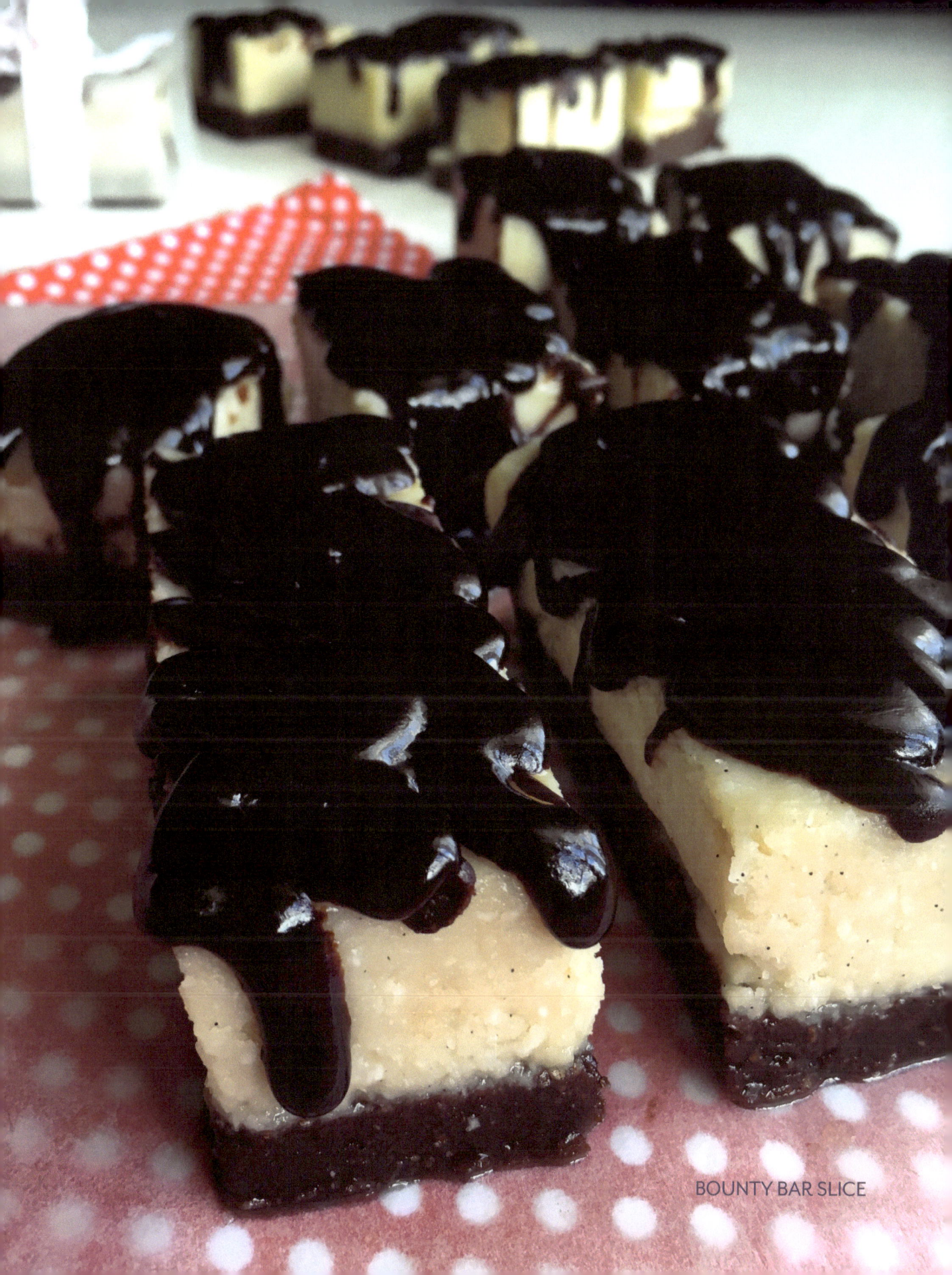

BOUNTY BAR SLICE

Lemon Slice

I've reinvented the old fashioned Lemon Slice to be grain free and vegan without losing any of its classic taste.

Chocolate is wonderful, but given the choice of a chocolate dessert or something fruity, I will usually go the fruity path. Given the choice of a fruit dessert that contains lemon, and lemon wins every time.

This is very lemony because I like my flavor to hit me like a truck. If you're a little subtler than I, add less rind.

Lacuma powder lends a sweet and citrusy flavor. It is a Peruvian fruit available from the health food store in a powder. Don't panic if you can't find it. I'm sure this works equally as well without it. This recipe is a great way to use up leftover almond pulp but if you don't have any, just use whole almonds and grind them in the food processor.

INGREDIENTS

Base

- » 1 cup almond pulp
- » 1 cup dates
- » 1 cup desiccated coconut
- » 3 tbs lemon rind (3 lemons)
- » 1/2 cup lemon juice (or juice of 2 lemons)
- » 2 tbs lacuma powder
- » 1 tsp vanilla paste
- » 1 tbs coconut oil or coconut paste

Topping

- » 1/2 cup coconut paste
- » 2 tbs lemon rind
- » juice of 1 lemon
- » 2 - 3 tbs rice malt syrup (I used 2 tbs and then 1 microspoon of stevia)

METHOD

Base

Blend all ingredients in food processor and press into a tray lined with baking paper.

Topping

Blend these ingredients in a food processor. Pour this gorgeous topping onto the base and smooth with a spatula before setting in the fridge.

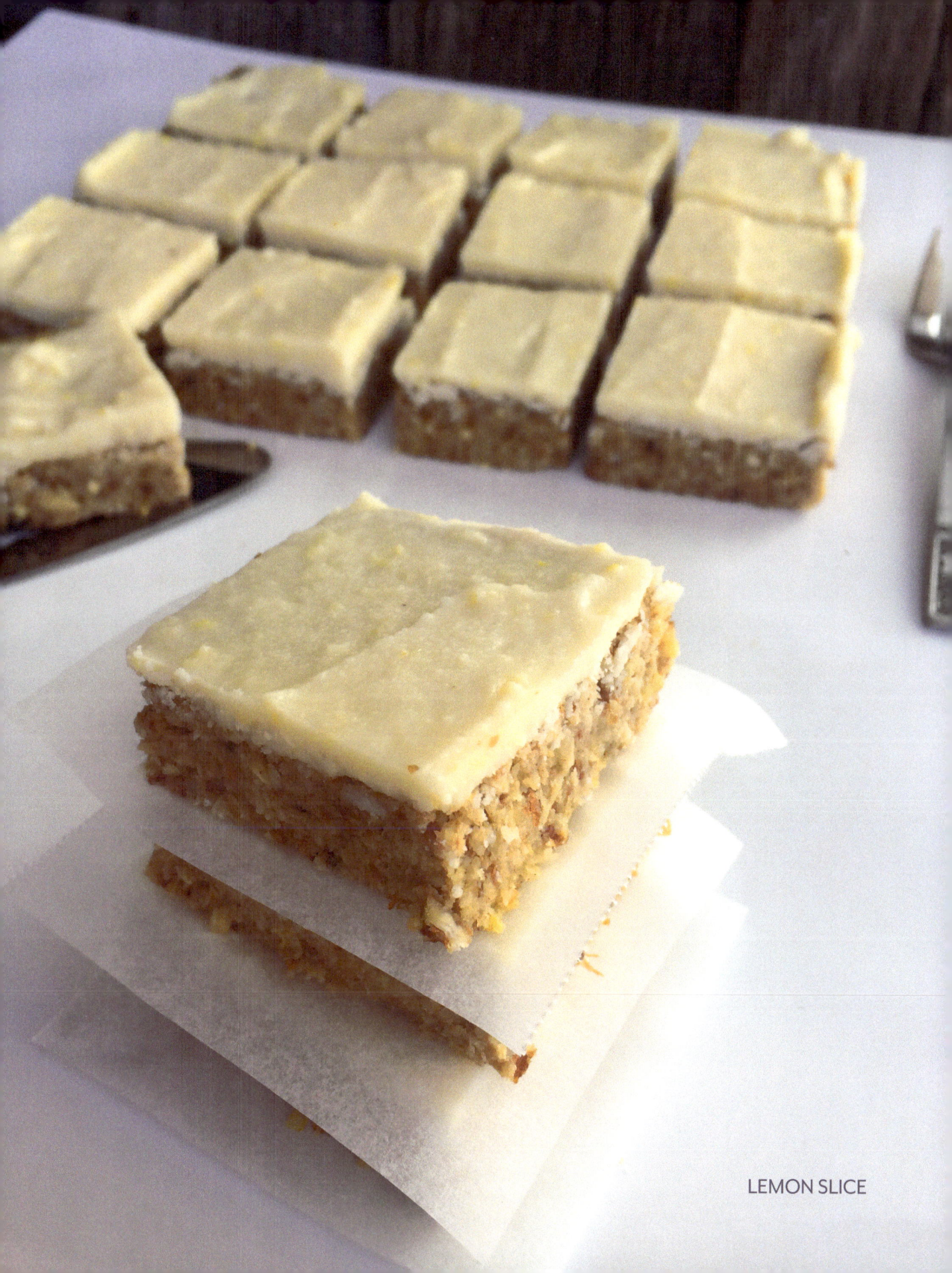

LEMON SLICE

Choc Peanut Butter Protein Slice

If you love peanut butter and chocolate, then this is your thing. I've added the linseeds (flaxseeds) for a bit of crunch factor and brain boost - think Omega 3s. Chia seeds and protein powder up the protein hit. Perfect for after your workout session. Roll them into balls or press them into bars. They keep perfectly in the freezer for an emergency snack and are great for lunch boxes.

INGREDIENTS

- 1 cup raw peanut butter
- 1/3 cup raw cashews soaked
- 1/3 raw almonds soaked
- 2/3 cup dates
- 1/3 cup desiccated coconut
- 1/4 cup chia seeds
- 1/4 cup flaxseeds
- 2 tbs raw cacao powder
- 2 scoops vanilla protein powder (I used vanilla Sunwarrior)
- salt

METHOD

Blend nuts, add cacao and dates and continue blending. Add peanut butter and coconut. Blend in the remaining ingredients. Shape into balls or spread into a biscuit tray. Refrigerate until set.

NOTE:

If you don't pre-soak your nuts, it may be a little dry, so add some water to help mix in the protein powder.

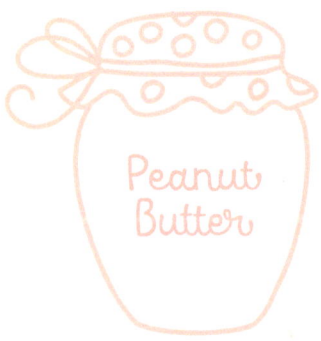

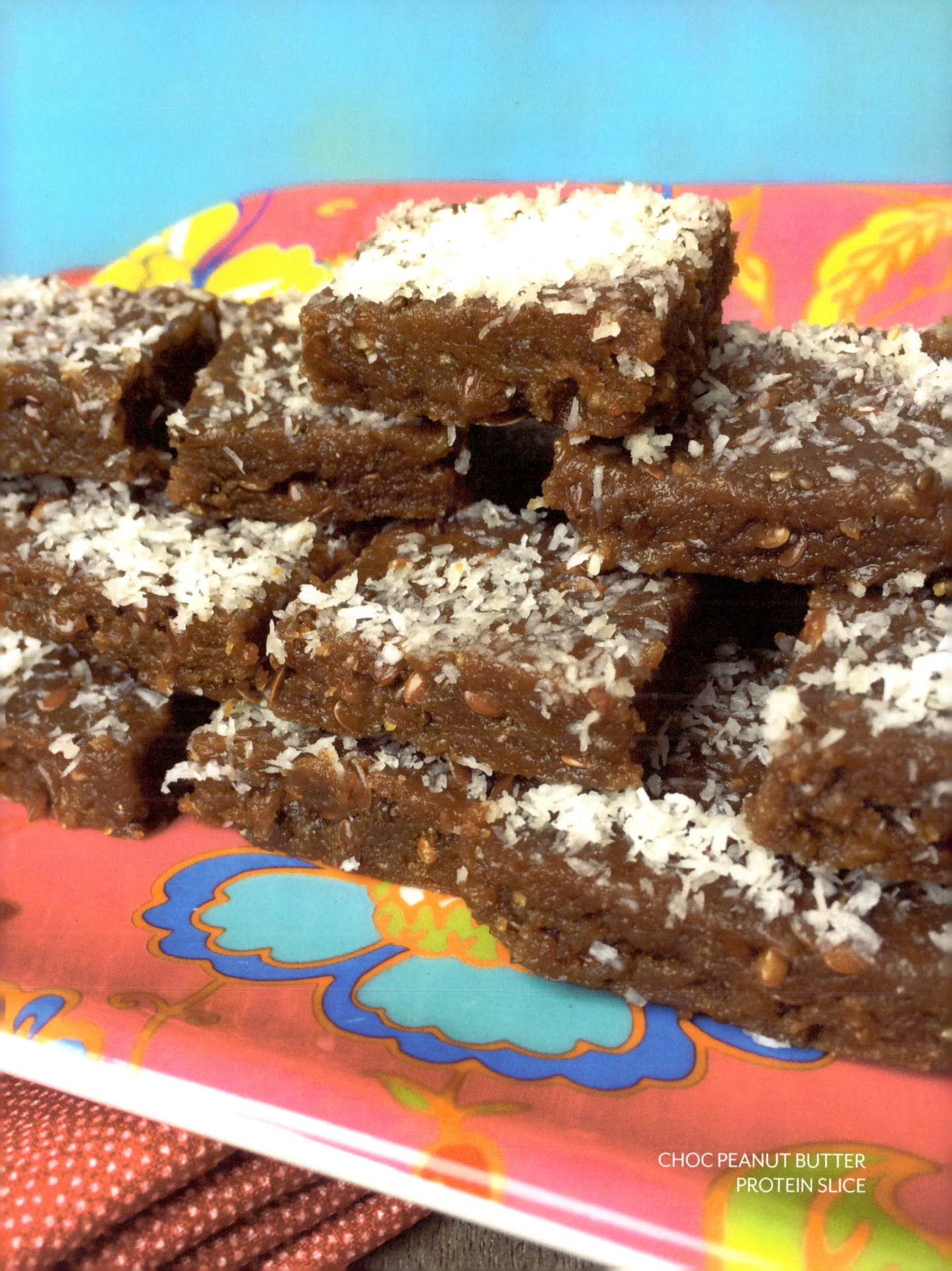

CHOC PEANUT BUTTER PROTEIN SLICE

Peanut Butter Protein Balls

This is a scrumptious way to get a protein hit and satisfy those afternoon chocolate cravings. I've used pure peanut butter from the health food store. They grind the nuts into a paste in store, and apart from it being pure peanuts with nothing else added, it is also cheaper than buying a branded concoction. I came upon this recipe because I had some vanilla protein powder I wanted to use up. Peanut butter has quite a strong flavor so I knew it would disguise the raw vegan protein powder.

INGREDIENTS

Peanut Ball – Makes 18 (if you don't snack)

- 1 cup pure peanut butter
- 1/4 cup coconut paste
- 1/2 cup pure maple syrup
- 40g or 1 scoop vanilla vegan protein powder (more if you like)
- 1/4 tsp pink salt

Chocolate Coating

- 1/2 cup melted cacao butter or 100g
- 1/2 cup raw cacao powder
- 1/4 cup maple syrup
- vanilla stevia drops (for optional extra sweetening)
- 3 Medicine Flower white chocolate drops (Extra bonus but optional)

METHOD

Peanut Ball

Blend all ingredients in a food processor and add salt to taste. Squeeze the mixture into a ball with your hands. It should hold together nicely. If you think it can hold more protein powder, then add another tablespoon. If you think it needs to be sweeter, than add some vanilla stevia drops. Don't add more syrup. Roll into balls and place on a tray lined with baking paper. Freeze while you make the chocolate.

Chocolate Coating

After melting the cacao butter by placing a glass or metal bowl in a bowl of hot water, stir in all ingredients. If you need it sweeter, then boost with vanilla stevia drops, but don't add more maple syrup as it will be too runny. Use a fork to dip the peanut balls into the chocolate. Allow the excess chocolate to drip off into the bowl then slide onto a baking paper lined tray with the push of a toothpick.

Refrigerate or freeze until chocolate is set. I photographed mine on a hot day but it will make a nice smooth glossy coating. There is enough chocolate for a double dipping.

 If you are short on time or don't think you want to mess around with double dipping, then place all balls into the chocolate bowl to coat. Then pour out into a deep baking tray lined with baking paper. Spread the balls out and refrigerate. Cut when set. Enjoy.

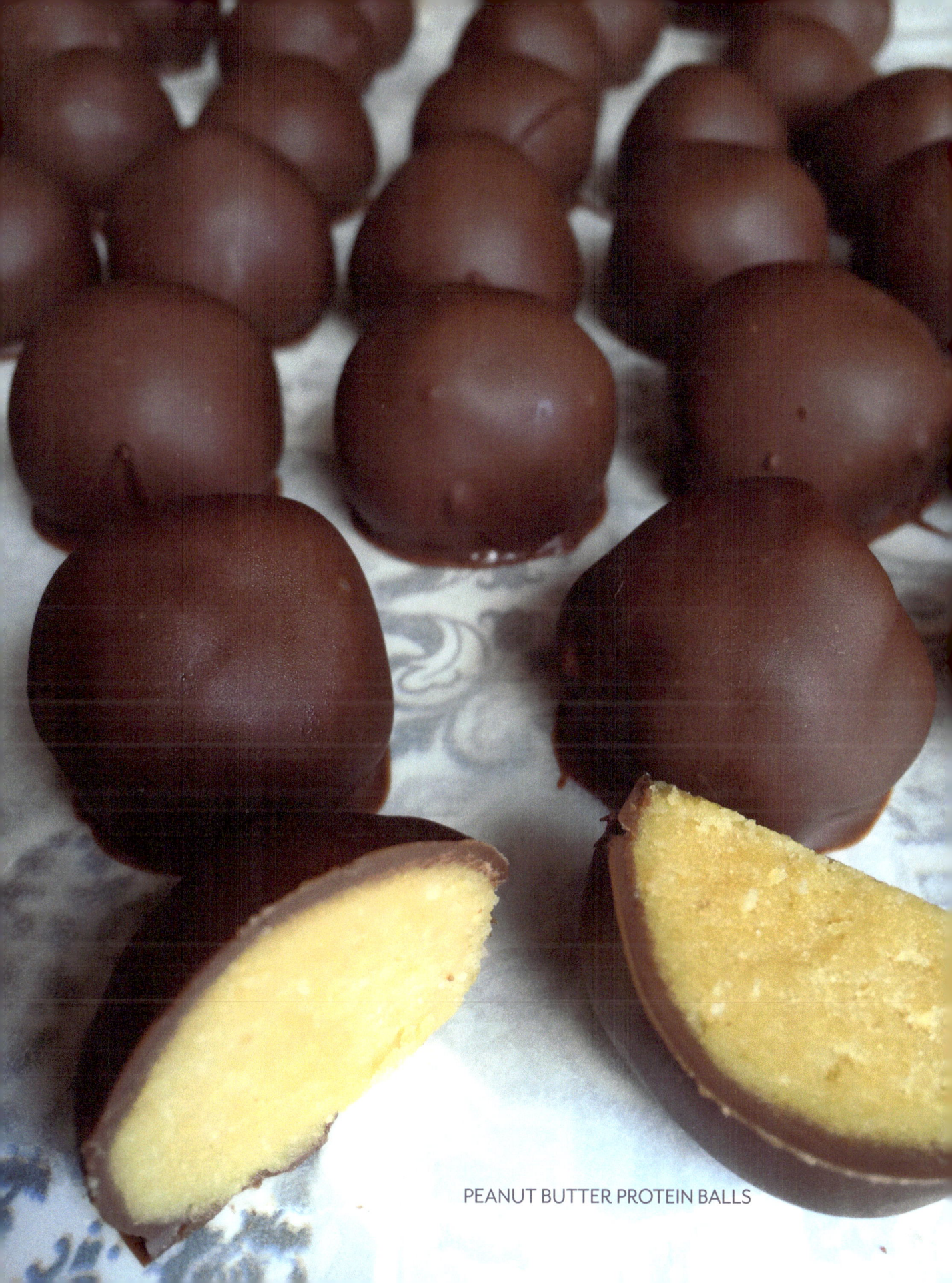

PEANUT BUTTER PROTEIN BALLS

Ginger and Turmeric Energy Balls

The combination of turmeric and ginger make this an anti-inflammatory power house.

I made these for my mother because she loves tahini, she loves ginger and... Well, everyone can benefit from the health benefits of the key ingredients.

INGREDIENTS

- » 1/2 cup almonds
- » 1/2 cup cashews
- » 1/2 cup desiccated coconut
- » 1 cup dried apricots
- » 1/4 cup grated fresh ginger (more or less depending on the potency of your ginger)
- » 1/4 cup tahini
- » 2 – 3 tsp turmeric powder
- » 1 tbs orange or lemon rind (or both)
- » 1 tbs chia seeds
- » 1 tbs lacuma powder

METHOD

Blend all dry ingredients together. Add the ginger and apricots. Continue blending until the mixture forms a doughy ball. Roll into small balls and coat in additional chia seeds and coconut. Makes 20 balls.

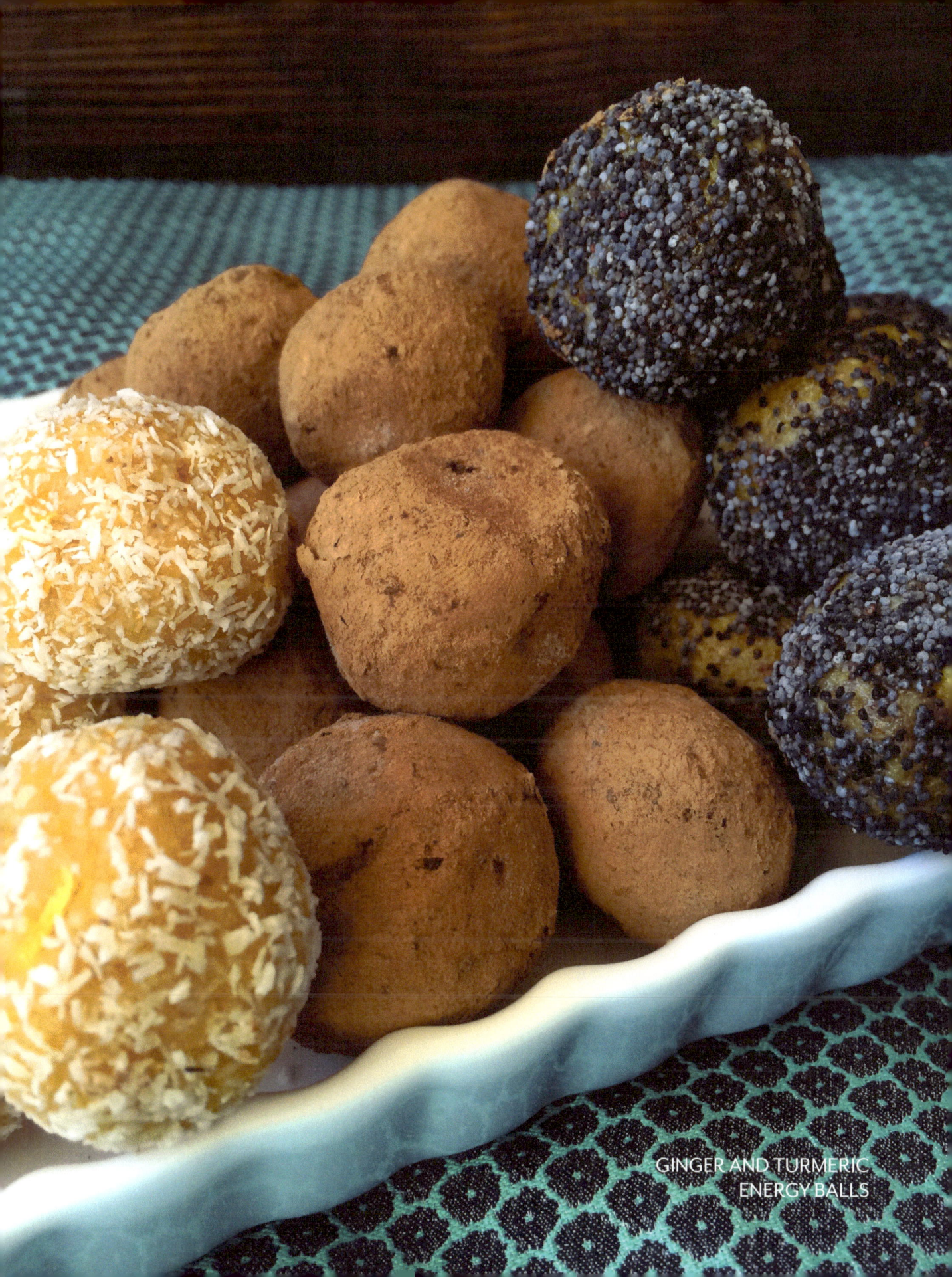

GINGER AND TURMERIC
ENERGY BALLS

Pumpkin Pie

If you like a toffee tasting pumpkin pie, then you will love this healthy version.

This is a perfect recipe for using left over almond pulp after making your own almond milk. Tip: When you make your almond milk throw in the vanilla bean when blending with water, then once the nuts are strained and squeezed, the ground vanilla pod will be left behind with the nuts.

INGREDIENTS

Base

- 1 1/2 cups almond pulp
- 1 whole vanilla bean (blitzed in a spice grinder) or 1 tsp of vanilla paste or 1 tbs vanilla essence
- 1 packed cup of dates
- 1/4 cup coconut oil
- crackle of pink salt

Pumpkin Filling

- 2 1/2 cups cooked and mashed pumpkin (roasted is best)
- 1 cup of almonds or 1 cup of almond butter (only use whole almonds if you have a powerful food processor that can turn them into paste)
- 3/4 cup lacuma powder
- 1/4 cup coconut oil (melted)
- 1/2 cup coconut paste (melted)
- 2 tsp cinnamon powder
- 2 tsp nutmeg powder
- 1/4 cup maple syrup
- salt on top

METHOD

Base

Process all ingredients in a high-powered food processor until it sticks together in a ball of dough when pressed. Line a fan pan with baking paper. (I like to trace out a circle and cut it to fit the base exactly.) Press the dough down uniformly and line the sides to form a pie crust. Refrigerate while you make the filling.

Pumpkin Filling

Blend almonds first until smooth. Add remaining ingredients and process for a few minutes, stopping to scrape down the sides. Spoon filling on top of pie crust and allow to set in the refrigerator for several hours until firm. Top with pistachio nuts.

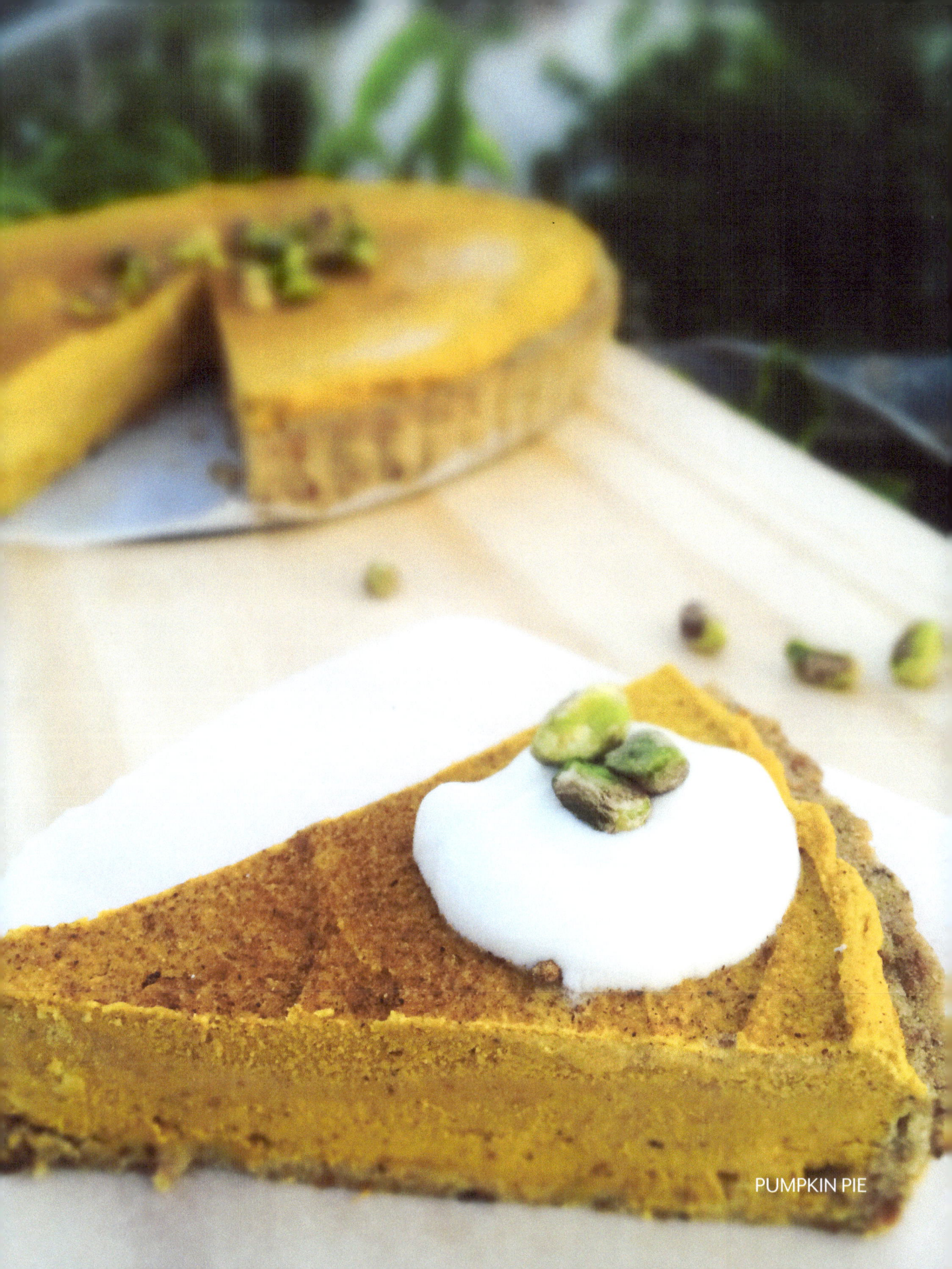

PUMPKIN PIE

Salted Caramel Chocolate Brownie

Glossy chocolate, gooey caramel and chewy brownie. You're going to love this.

Rest assured, this goodness is raw, vegan, dairy-free, gluten-free, grain-free, sugar-free, and still a 'knock your socks off' kind of chocolatey dessert.

INGREDIENTS

Base

- 2 1/2 cups walnuts
- 3 cups dates
- 1/2 cup raw cacao

Salted Caramel Layer

- 1/2 cup pure coconut cream
- 1/2 cup dates or 8 large Medjool dates
- 1 tbs vanilla extract
- 1 tsp Maldon sea salt flakes

Chocolate topping

- 1/4 cup coconut oil melted
- 1/4 cup maple syrup
- 1/4 cup raw cacao powder
- 3 tbs coconut cream

METHOD

Base

Blend dry ingredients in food processor until crumbly. Add dates a few at a time and continue blending until gooey and chewy. Press evenly into a square baking tin lined with baking paper.

Salted Caramel Layer

Blend all ingredients in the small bowl of your food processor until creamy. Pour onto the chocolate base.

Chocolate topping

Mix the oil and cacao in a bowl first. Then add the cream and maple syrup. The maple may cause the chocolate to seize a little. This is useful so it becomes firm. Spread the chocolate over the caramel with the back of a spoon or a palette knife. Refrigerate until set. Slice into squares.

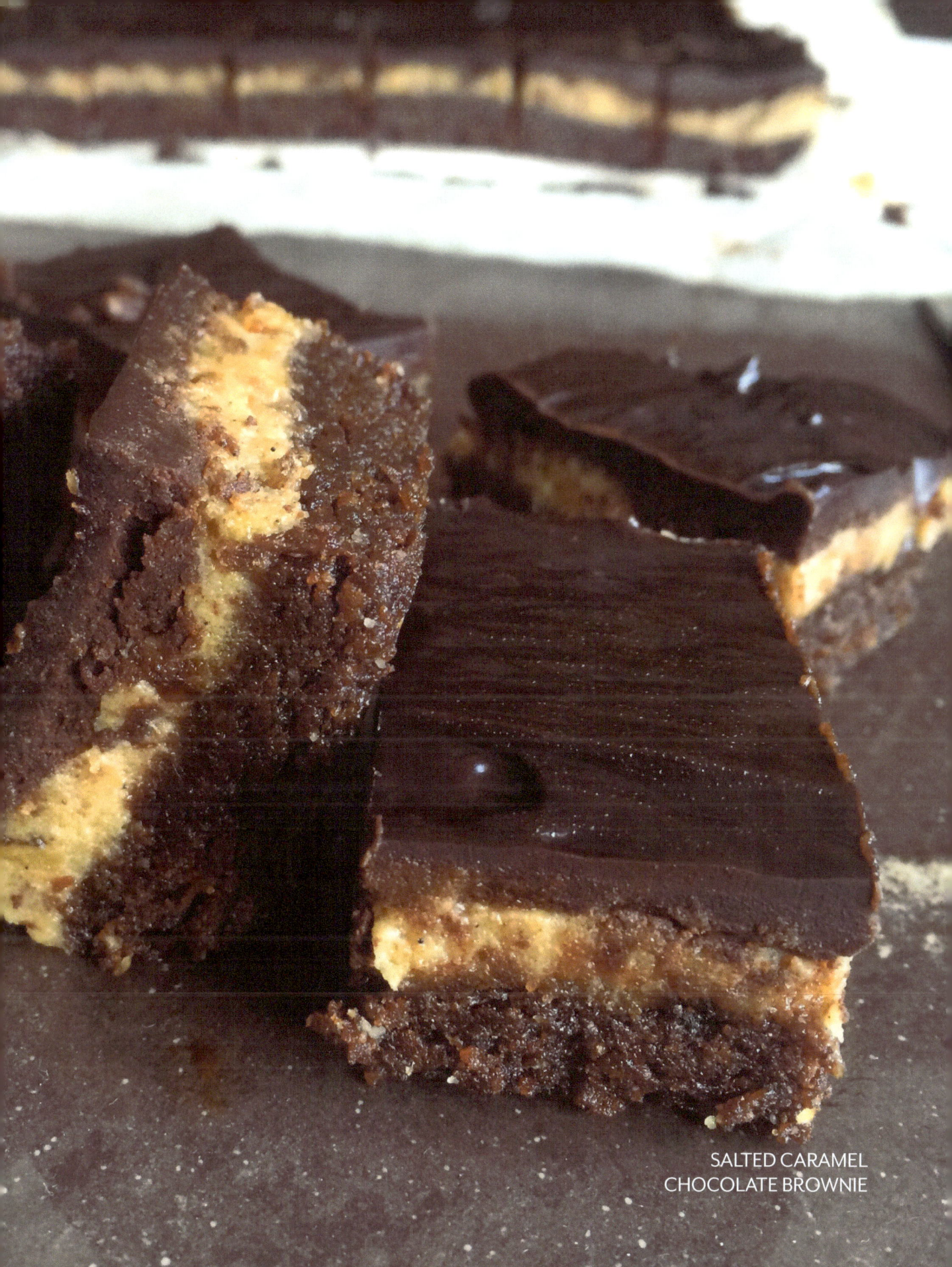

SALTED CARAMEL
CHOCOLATE BROWNIE

Rafaello Bites

I adore receiving a box of Rafaellos. But the trouble is I devour these coco-nutty bliss balls in one sitting. During one such occasion I mused, 'There must be a way to make a healthy version,' and there is. The crunchy wafer is absent but there is a crunch on a central almond and a bite through a creamy white chocolate shell. Munch down on sweet vanilla infused coconut and you will be in heaven. I've used skewers for ease of dipping and I thought the sewers made them look as cute as cake pops. You could try toothpicks or just a fork.

INGREDIENTS

- 1 1/2 cup desiccated coconut
- 1/4 cup 100% coconut cream.
- 1/4 cup Rice malt syrup
- 1/4 cup coconut paste
- 1 tsp vanilla extract
- 15 whole almonds

White chocolate coating

- 1/2 cup cacao butter (melted)
- 1/4 cup cashews soaked
- 1/4 cup maple syrup
- 4 white chocolate essence drops or 1 tsp of vanilla extract
- 1/2 cup Coconut for dusting

METHOD

Blend all ingredients (except almonds) in a food processor until well combined. Roll into balls and insert an almond into the centre. Roll between palms again until smooth. Place balls on a tray lined with baking paper and freeze while you make the white chocolate. If you are going to use skewers then insert them now.

White chocolate coating

Blend cashews in the small bowl of the food processor, and pour in melted cacao butter. Process until smooth and glossy. Pour in maple syrup and continue processing. Dip coconut balls in white chocolate and return to freezer to set. Make a second dip into the white chocolate but this time roll in a little desiccated coconut and then place on tray and refrigerate. Once set, eat them or drizzle on more chocolate.

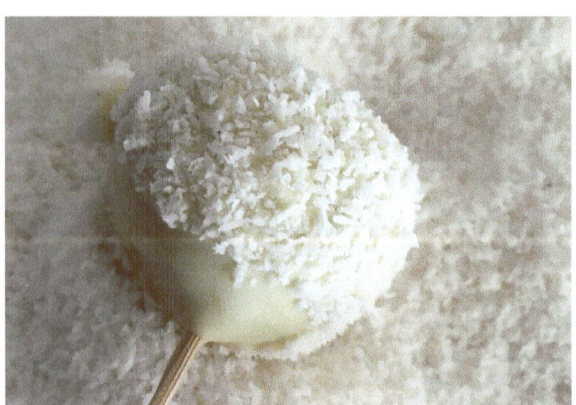

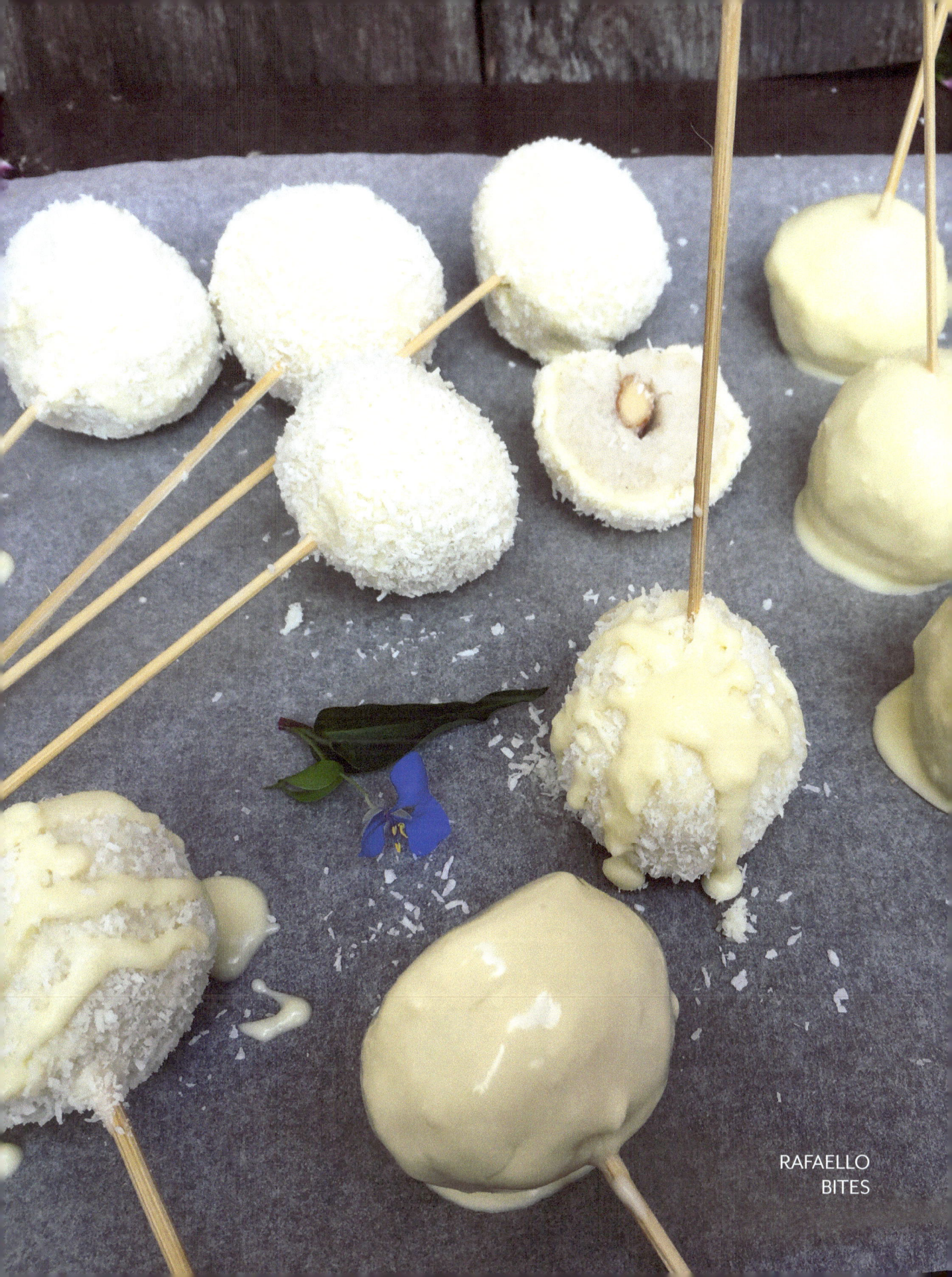

RAFAELLO BITES

White Christmas Slice

A traditional white Christmas slice is made from powdered milk, icing sugar, Copha, dried fruit and rice bubbles. I've recreated this Christmas favourite into a clean version without the milk and sugar. It tastes like a white chocolate fruit cake, but don't wait until Christmas to try it.

INGREDIENTS

- 1/2 cup melted cacao butter
- 1/2 cup dried apricots chopped
- 1 cup dried fruit (1/3 cup cranberries, 1/3 cup sultanas, 1/3 cup Goji berries)
- 1 cup desiccated coconut
- 1 cup cashews
- 1/2 cup buckinis (activated buckwheat) optional

METHOD

Melt cacao butter in a jug placed inside a bowl of hot water. Grind cashews in a spice grinder until flour is formed or you can use 3/4 cup cashew butter. Mix all ingredients together in a bowl. Press into a tin lined with baking paper. Refrigerate until set. Slice into squares.

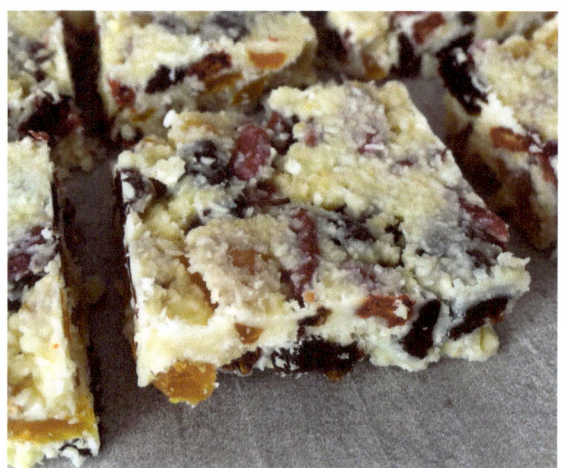

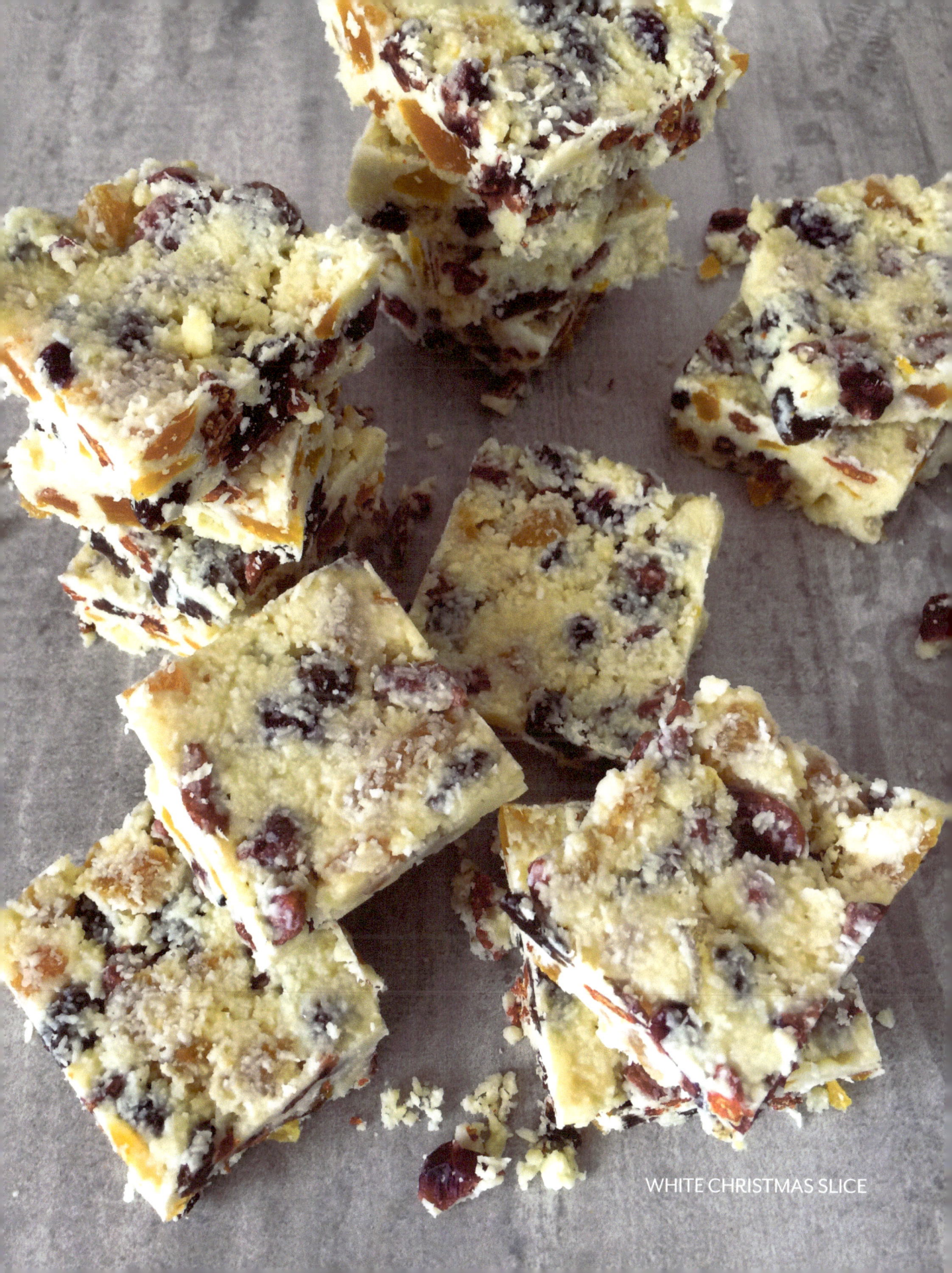
WHITE CHRISTMAS SLICE

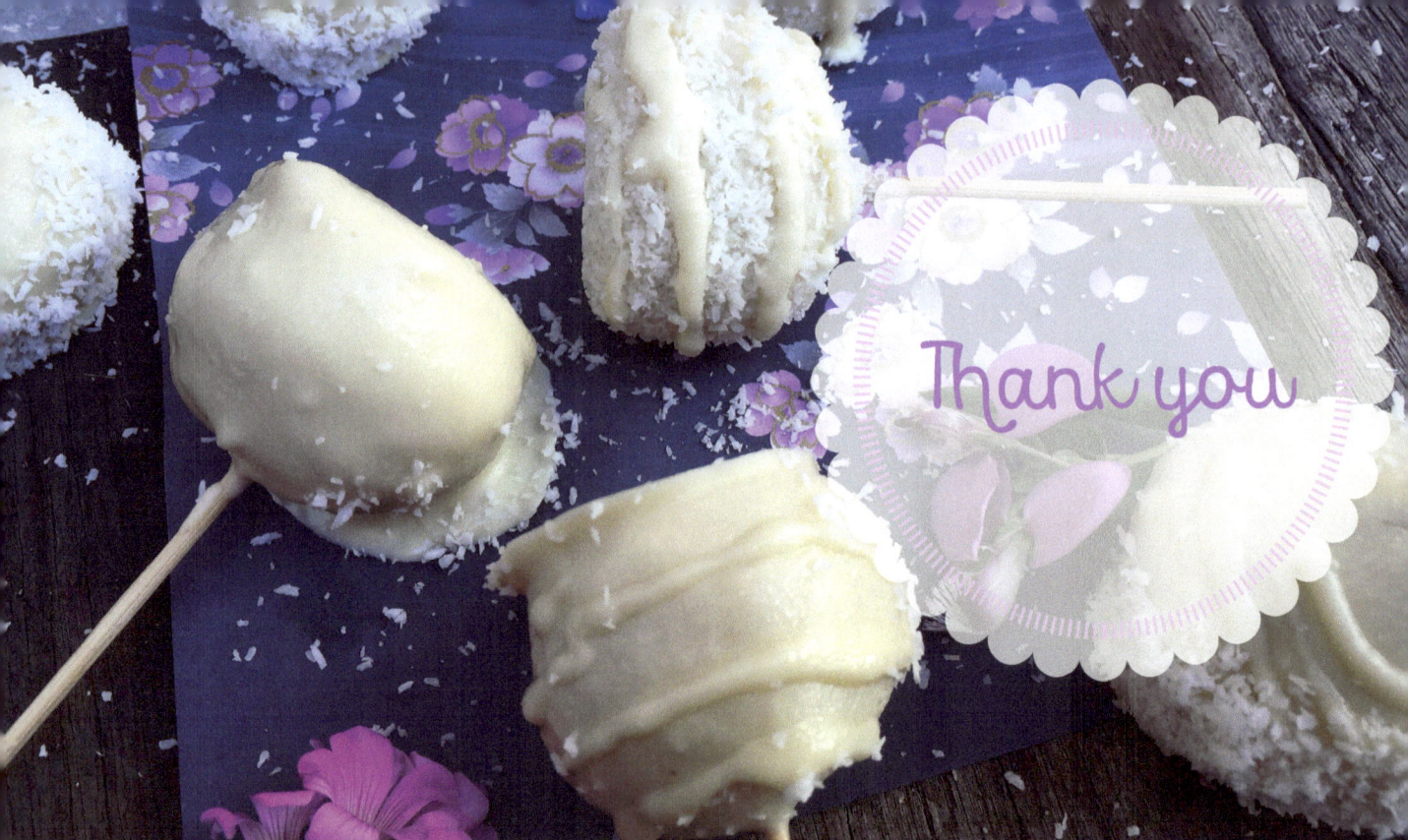

A book is not possible without the help of many people.

Thank you to Lisa Valuyskaya for her creative design skills. Lisa not only transformed my notes into a beautiful book, but she was able to translate my often befuddled instructions.

Many thanks for Chantal Darcy, my beautiful sister who helped formulate this book and my previous book, The Great Uncooking. She sifted through hundreds of photos and organised my chaotic mind, giving me 'to do' lists to break down this daunting task into manageable bits. I'm especially grateful for her miraculous recovery from leukaemia last year. Without her this book would still be pages of messy handwritten notes scattered all over my desk.

I'm grateful to my mother, who taught me how to throw together random ingredients with delicious results. She too, could never follow a recipe, instead substituting with what she had or amplifying flavour. For her, having 8 different vegetables in a meal made a great dinner. Alice Prigoone is truly the mother of invention. She also taste tested just about everything in this book, providing valuable feedback.

Thank you to Marj Osborne for her expert editing, efficiency and eye for detail. Without her, I probably would have misspelt my own name.

Lastly, thank you to you. The more people who embrace a healthy way of eating, the easier it is to live this way.

About the author

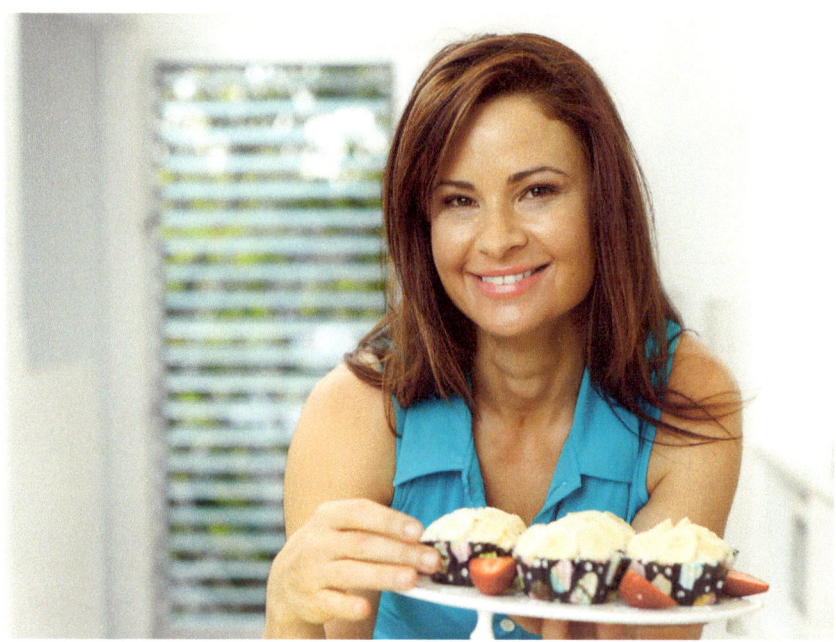

Natalie and food have long been synonymous. After a foray into reality television with the first season of My Restaurant Rules (2003) and her restaurant Mylk (My little kitchen), Natalie has now become a passionate speaker on raw food. She is also the author of "The Great Uncooking: Real Food|Raw Food" (2014) a chunky detox bible packed full of healthy raw food recipes.

Since her early teens, Natalie has appeared in over 130 television commercials from Johnson & Johnson, to Sprite and Holden,

Her film credits include working as a picture double for the James Cameron film Sanctum, and an extra on films such as Mental.

Natalie loves random world travel, has scaled the Himalayas, jumped from a plane and travelled the world as an Emirates flight attendant.

When not experimenting in the kitchen, Natalie works as a yoga instructor and high school teacher. If you happen to drop into her house she will make sure you don't leave without first sampling some homemade dessert.

Index

A
Almond milk ... 14

B
Banana Almond Choc Coated Fudge ... 86
Banana and Mango Hemp Cookies ... 104
Banana Strawberry Layered Cheesecake ... 46
Blueberry Pikelets ... 92
Bounty Bar Slice ... 108
Brandy Black Forest Ice-creams ... 40

BREAKFAST DESSERTS ... 91
Blueberry Pikelets ... 92
Chocolate Buckini Muesli with Almond Milk ... 94
Green Chia Pudding ... 100
Pear and Raspberry Chia Pudding ... 96
Strawberry Coconut Chia Pudding ... 98

C
Chaimisu ... 66

CHEESECAKES ... 43
Banana Strawberry Layered Cheesecake ... 46
Chaimisu ... 66
Cherry Lemon Cheesecake ... 64
Chocolate Ganache Cakes with Orange Segments ... 48
Lemon, Lavender and Blueberry Cheesecakes ... 56
Lime Chocolate Cheesecake ... 50
Mango Lychee Cheesecakes ... 52
Raspberry and Pomegranate Mini Cheesecakes ... 60
Salted Caramel Cream Cake ... 62
Spiced Apple Cakes with Cream ... 70
White Chocolate Cheesecake with Strawberries ... 44
White Chocolate Cherry Cheesecake ... 54

White Chocolate Mango Cheesecake ... 56
Cherry Lemon Cheesecake ... 64
Choc Peanut Butter Protein Slice ... 112

CHOCOLATE & FUDGE ... 73
Banana Almond Choc Coated Fudge ... 86
Chocolate Fudge ... 84
Chocolate Mousse Parfait ... 88
Chocolate Peppermint Slice ... 80
Maple Walnut Fudge ... 82
Mint Chocolate Thins ... 74
The Chocolate Road ... 78
White Chocolate Chunk ... 76

Chocolate Buckini Muesli with Almond Milk ... 94
Chocolate Fudge ... 84
Chocolate Ganache Cakes with Orange Segments ... 48
Chocolate Mousse Parfait ... 88
Chocolate Peppermint Slice ... 80
Chocolate Rosemary Ice-cream ... 34
Coconut Mango Lime Ice-cream ... 30
Coconut Vanilla Banana Ice-cream ... 24

COOKIES, SLICES & ENERGY BALLS ... 103
Banana and Mango Hemp Cookies ... 104
Bounty Bar Slice ... 108
Choc Peanut Butter Protein Slice ... 112
Ginger and Turmeric Energy Balls ... 116
Lemon Slice ... 110
Peanut Butter Protein Balls ... 114
Pumpkin Pie ... 118
Rafaello Bites ... 122
Raw Iced VoVo ... 106
Salted Caramel Chocolate Brownie ... 120
White Christmas Slice ... 124

G

Ginger and Turmeric Energy Balls 116
Green Chia Pudding 100

I

ICE-CREAMS 19

    Brandy Black Forest Ice-creams 40
    Chocolate Rosemary Ice-cream 34
    Coconut Vanilla Banana Ice-cream 24
    Coconut Mango Lime Ice-cream 30
    Lavender Blueberry Ice-cream 36
    Mango and Coconut Yoghurt Ice-cream Bars 28
    Mint Chocolate Ice-cream Blocks with Chlorella 26
    Peanut Butter Cup Ice-cream 38
    Raspberry Coconut Ice-cream Blocks 22
    Raspberry Tamarind Sorbet 32
    Strawberry 20

L

Lavender Blueberry Ice-cream 36
Lemon, Lavender and Blueberry Cheesecakes 56
Lemon Slice 110
Lime Chocolate Cheesecake 50

M

Mango and Coconut Yoghurt Ice-cream Bars 28
Mango Lychee Cheesecakes 52
Maple Walnut Fudge 82
Milk, Almond 14
Mint Chocolate Ice-cream Blocks with Chlorella 26
Mint Chocolate Thins 74

P

Peanut Butter Cup Ice-cream 38
Peanut Butter Protein Balls 114
Pear and Raspberry Chia Pudding 96
Pumpkin Pie 118

R

Rafaello Bites 122
Raspberry and Pomegranate Mini Cheesecakes 60
Raspberry Coconut Ice-cream Blocks 22
Raspberry Tamarind Sorbet 32
Raw Iced VoVo 106

S

Salted Caramel Chocolate Brownie 120
Salted Caramel Cream Cake 62
Spiced Apple Cakes with Cream 70
Strawberry Coconut Chia Pudding 98
Strawberry Ice-cream 20

T

The Chocolate Road 78

W

White Chocolate Cheesecake with Strawberries 44
White Chocolate Cherry Cheesecake 54
White Chocolate Chunk 76
White Chocolate Mango Cheesecake 56
White Christmas Slice 124

www.ingramcontent.com/pod-product-compliance
Lightning Source LLC
Chambersburg PA
CBHW041123300426
44113CB00002B/43